How to Back up Without Giving up

How to Back up Without Giving up

Stephen Baron

Writers Club Press
New York Lincoln Shanghai

How to Back up Without Giving up

Writers Club Press
an imprint of iUniverse, Inc.

For information address:
iUniverse, Inc.
2021 Pine Lake Road, Suite 100
Lincoln, NE 68512
www.iuniverse.com

ISBN: 0-595-25907-3 (pbk)
ISBN: 0-595-65424-X (cloth)

Printed in the United States of America

For Nancy J. Havernick, M.D.

Contents

Preface

This book fulfills a promise I made fifteen or so years ago. When I was hospitalized with an MS exacerbation (attack), I received a treatment of physical therapy daily. I felt so buoyed by the workout, I asked the director of the Department where I could connect with a good physical therapist. He responded,

"You don't need a physical therapist. You have a great attitude, and that alone is more than half the battle. You're your own best physical therapist. You ought to share your attitude with other people."

"I don't do support groups," I responded, "but I'll write a book which conveys my attitude."

Thus the genesis of this book. Directly or indirectly I have worked on it ever since. My deepest hope is that it might help others with MS pursue a fulfilling life. MS, I firmly believe, is not the end of life. Rather, it simply makes leading a full life more difficult. Do I enjoy having MS? Not a bit, but I've never used it as an excuse for withdrawing from life. Technology has made life more accessible for the handicapped. That this entire book was composed using a voice input computer is testament to advances in technology.

As well, I hope that it might help others who know an MS sufferer. Everyone suffers a handicap of one sort or another, from arthritis to tinnitus. Each limits life in its own particular way. Learning how to pursue a complete life, illness, notwithstanding, is a challenge everyone faces. I hope that by understanding MS better, people will be able to lead fuller, more complete lives.

Acknowledgments

Many individuals assisted me along the way. Without implying a greater or lesser debt, I will simply list them: Jeff Carmen, Jon and Randi Herskowitz, JoHannah Laurie, Cindy Fields, John K. Wolfe, Efrain Perez, Ron Loewenstein, Alison Bert, Carol Rosenberg, Diane Hainesworth, Sr. Mary Brian Bole, Aimee Friedman, and Billie Brannock. Their help has been invaluable. My apologies to all those whom I have forgotten to thank.

I cannot close without thanking my daughters, Alexis and Miriam, and most of all my wife Nancy J. Havernick., M.D.

Stephen Baron
Syracuse, NY
February, 2001

Introduction

Multiple Sclerosis is a debilitating disease that can render life miserable. Translated precisely, MS, or 'many scars', is thought to be an auto-immune illness. So named because it leaves scars on the brain and central nervous system that can be seen on autopsy. Today, the scars, or plaques, as the medical community refers to them, are visible on a computer-generated picture of the brain. This is what an MRI (magnetic resonance imaging) machine does. First it magnetically aligns all the body's molecules along a vertical axis, then generates another strong magnetic field at a right angle to the first, having the effect of bending all the molecules over. Last, the horizontal magnetic field is turned off allowing the molecules to return to their original vertical alignment. Different molecules emit electrical impulses in this process of realignment. A 'picture' of the brain is constructed from these impulses. This non-invasive diagnostic device is little short of amazing.

The immune (disease fighting) system we each have is composed of two parts: killer cells which attack a foreign agent that invades the body, and regulator cells that tell the killer cells when to attack and when to stand down. What happens in MS is that the killer cells mistake one's own body for an invading agent they eat away at the myelin sheath coating the nerves. After many years, the damage extends to the nerves themselves. The best analogy I have heard is that it's like eating the insulation off an electric cord on a lamp or appliance. The result is a short circuit. In our nervous system, a similar thing occurs: the impulses from the brain get to the muscles more slowly, or not at all. Hence, paralysis, partial or total. Most often, the legs are affected because the pathways in the central nervous system, through which the impulses controlling them travel, are the longest in the body making them most accessible to damage.

Frequently, if not constantly, MS challenges our mental and physical existence. My entire enterprise in writing this book is to teach MS sufferers how it is possible to pursue a fulfilling, satisfying life despite MS. More, I believe we can all make a contribution to the betterment of humanity.

The progress of my case of MS is not unusual. When first diagnosed in March 1982, I could walk or swim as far as I wanted. Three or four years later, the walks of several miles yielded to a stroll around the block, until even that required the assistance of forearm [Canadian] crutches. The day it took me an hour to walk half a mile using crutches, I announced to my wife, "Now is the time for a [wheel] chair." Little did I think I would ever say those words. As for swimming, I relied on the assistance of children's water wings positioned behind my knees to keep my legs afloat.

There is a tendency to think our case is the worst imaginable, that nobody has suffered as we have. But, this is clearly false. MS is not unique. Actually, I do not believe it is any worse than any other chronic illness. What distinguishes it is that it is ours. Nobody can fully appreciate the extent or depth of our plight. It is unreasonable to expect that of anyone else.

Currently, the government estimates that over 50 million people are afflicted with a chronic illness. From bursitis to varicose veins, angina to osteoporosis, both rich and poor alike suffer. When we are no longer free to do as we please, when our diets are restricted in undesirable, and sometimes painful ways, how do we go on?

My response has been neither to capitulate nor to overpower the illness. Whether from pride or foolishness, I simply refuse to do the former, and am too small to entertain the idea of the latter. Fashioned by the challenge of seeing my independence slowly, yet relentlessly, taken from me, I have learned to live within the confines established by

MS. Rational acceptance and reasonable management have guided me in living. These two principles require neither great physical prowess nor capitulation. They can be applied to any chronic illness, and hold out the prospect of leading a full life.

Returning to the perfect health, I realized, was not one of my options. No amount of trying, crying, hissing, spitting, or cussing would accomplish that. I would simply have to accept my fate. Even the strongest athlete cannot escape the toll that MS exacts. Strength alone is not the key.

Having once accepted the reality of the situation, the next step was figuring out how to manage my new circumstances. For the walking, I really wanted and needed mobility. Hence, a wheelchair was in order. Liking the idea of a wheelchair was not one of my options. If I wanted to remain independent and mobile, a wheelchair was the only reasonable choice. For swimming, as I said above, children's arm floats affixed behind my knees was an innovation that still impresses physical therapists. In both cases the solution was the same: discovering a new means to the same end, albeit qualified by the limitations of the situation.

Are my solutions perfect? Of course not. But, given my circumstance, I realize that I cannot measure satisfaction by the standard of a person in perfect health. Rather, having accepted the curse of MS, the meaning of satisfaction had to be fashioned anew. According to the new reality of a life with chronic illness, yes, I am satisfied.

To be sure everything here will not apply to everyone. Indeed, even every case of MS, even those that act clinically alike, are not identical. Each is unique because every individual suffering it is unique. Nevertheless, the broad principles involved in confronting MS are similar: rational acceptance and reasonable management.

My message is not inspirational. Rather, it is an approach to living that requires diligence, patience, and commitment to one's own happiness. Applied judiciously to all the special situations that result from MS, they can make it possible to live a full and satisfying life.

1

Presentation

We begin thinking about our health only when some grievous illness befalls us, when an illness 'presents'. Fair enough, but when is that? It has been said that we all get thirty free years. This number is somewhat arbitrary. It could be more, it could be less, but that is of little consequence. The fact remains that in our early years we all take our health for granted.

Witness young people. They act as if they are immortal. Why should we expect otherwise from people for whom thirty is old, forty is well beyond the pale, and fifty is definitely over the hill? So too is it any wonder that most violent crimes are committed by people who do not know what illness is, let alone death? Or, that rioting is done primarily by those under the age of 25?

I recall the way I could ignore, even abuse, my body when I was young. What I consumed, be it healthy, unhealthy, or positively dangerous was irrelevant because I knew that the next day I would be my old self again. I recall a professional football player observing that in his early years he could recover from Sunday's injuries on Monday. With each passing year, he found that recovery took a day longer. By the end of his career he could never fully recover. Rather than play in constant pain, he decided it was time to retire.

My students thought nothing of drinking too much, sleeping too little, and generally taking their health for granted. Is there any other way to explain their cavalier attitude about smoking, drinking, or AIDS?

"Oh, that's something someone else will get."

Likewise, lung cancer is not an illness they fear.

"I'd rather die happy than stop smoking."

Has there ever been a victim of lung cancer who has not regretted smoking?

No, those are the carefree years. The folly of youth is to believe that we are invulnerable.

As one great sage said, "The only problem with youth is that it is wasted on the young."

Exercising falls under a similar judgment. Consider, the age of the walkers or runners we ordinarily see on the streets. Rarely, are they adolescents. More often, they are in their 30s, 40s, or older. Likewise, health club members tend to be closer to middle age than adolescence. An exercise instructor told me that among students in her hundreds of classes, the vast majority are middle-aged.

To be fair, though, some of my students are aware of physical frailties. A few have parents with a debilitating disease. Others have grandparents in wheelchairs, while occasionally, there is the unfortunate student who is diagnosed with a chronic illness. They discover firsthand the need to begin life again qualified by the limits of the illness. I recall a student crying bitterly because she was diagnosed with Crohn's disease, an inflammatory disease of the digestive tract. On the eve of graduation, a few months away from marriage, and eager to begin a career as a school psychologist, she suddenly realized that all her plans had to be adjusted to the uncompromising demands of her illness. But, she is noteworthy, because her case is so unusual. Ordinarily, chronic illness is something associated with the elderly.

Then, one day, we discover something just isn't right. It could be a familiar symptom, a backache perhaps, or something more rarefied. In my case some friends noticed me dragging my right leg as I walked. But for their observations, I would likely have overlooked the problem for quite a long time. In typical fashion I would have dismissed it, or tried to shrug it off. The usual childhood illnesses aside, I had been healthy as a horse. There had been no broken bones, no extraordinary illnesses, or great physical challenges, nor had I been overweight. I was afflicted with the ordinary burden of environmental allergies. A nuisance, sure, but little more. The only time I had ever been in a hospital was as a visitor. At 30 years of age, I was the picture of health. Daily, I swam half a mile, or ran several miles. My diet, by all accounts, was healthy: vegetarian and low fat. I drank moderately, didn't smoke, and took no drugs. I felt well and looked fit. Regrettably, the juxtaposition of looking well, and being seriously constrained is quite common with MS.

As I often say, "Here I have this crummy disease, and I have nothing to show for it."

Having yet to discover this unfortunate truth, I blithely dismissed my symptom. Why not? There was no reason to suspect anything more than the ordinary muscle discomforts. After all, that's what my parents always said to do.

"No need to overreact. It will go away by itself if you just leave it alone."

This was generic advice that was appropriate to offer an adolescent excessively concerned with acne. Not surprisingly, it usually worked. No, just let the leg be. I was convinced it would get better on its own.

I recalled my grandmother's example. Questions of her health were a standing source of amusement among her grandchildren. Although we loved her dearly, none dared ask, 'How are you?' unless we were prepared to listen to a 20 minute discourse on all her maladies, imagined and real. She spent half her later years seeing a variety of doctors, and annually took a two-week vacation at the Massachusetts General Hospital. She would probably have died well short of her 96 birthday, I would say, had she not been so damned sick. My grandmother was a dear woman, and I will forever cherish my memories of her, but I never harbored any desire to emulate her example.

When benign neglect failed, I tried another favorite therapy: exercise. Rest might have been the wiser course of action, but, at my age and in my condition, that was tantamount to surrender. Concede was the last thing in the world I would have considered. In delicate times, moderation is recommended, but these were extraordinary circumstances that demanded extreme measures. Thus I initiated the most ill-conceived, poorly executed, and outrageously inappropriate regimen imaginable: running, walking, calisthenics, and swimming, all to the point of exhaustion.

"Exercise like there is no tomorrow. Yup, that'll fix it."

Not surprisingly, along with this mysterious symptom, I now hurt all over, and was embarrassed as well. Rest was not only the one thing I wanted to do, but the only thing I could do. Having rested to the point of utter boredom (at least 20 minutes), I turned to the next likely place for relief, over-the-counter drugs. The advertisements convey the impression that there is nothing they cannot fix—or at least relieve. But, I was unfamiliar with the gamut of remedies available. Besides, I had a general aversion to pills. I opted for the old standards: aspirin and acetaminophen. That I didn't understand the difference between them was irrelevant. Regardless, they turned out to be inadequate to the task.

How humbling to be forced to admit there are things beyond my control. What a terrifying discovery to be presented with a mystery that all the tried and true remedies would not fix. Oh, to suffer the blow to the male ego I insisted I never had. How could it be that 'Mr. Fiercely Independent' needed help? Horrors, the dreaded 'H' word. Little did I know that asking for help would become an everyday necessity for me. Only later did I discover that doing so without losing my dignity would be one of the most difficult challenges of my life.

As a last resort, I turned to friends, the place where I probably should have begun. Family would have done as well, but mine was hundreds of miles away. If my friends' infinite wisdom could not solve it, at least they could offer consolation. As in many cases, two heads, especially sympathetic ones, turn out to be better than one. If nothing else, they reinforce the invaluable lesson that none of us is either completely self-sufficient, or entirely alone.

However comforting, this was by no means a guarantee of a successful outcome. A teacher instructed me in this lesson through the story of Isadora Duncan and George Bernard Shaw. Though a great beauty and noted dancer, she was not known for her great intelligence. He, on the other hand, a famous playwright, was known for his great intellect, and particular homeliness. Isadora is said to have proposed a union in the hope that the progeny might have her beauty, and his brains. He respectfully declined on the grounds that the children might have her brains, and his looks.

The friend, whose counsel and comfort I solicited, presumed neither wisdom nor expertise. She pleaded ignorance of my symptoms. Instead, she promised to ask her psychiatrist about it. In a few days the answer came back: go have it checked out by a neurologist at the emergency room.

And, so I went. Not only was I completely unfamiliar with the emergency room, I'm not sure I knew what a neurologist does. I forgot that I had seen one when I was an undergraduate ten years earlier for symptoms that were the first foreshadowing of MS.

Upon entering the august facility, memories of 'Quiet Hospital Zone' came to mind. Reality quickly dashed my memories. Anyone who has had occasion to visit an emergency room at almost any hospital, at almost any hour of the day or night, can testify that it is a bee-hive of activity. Rarely are they sedate places.

Timidly, I approached the receptionist who seemed to be in charge, and explained what brought me there. Looking at the assembly of walking wounded, I felt a little sheepish for not having any visible signs for my visit. Not one to doubt my word, the harried receptionist inquired about enough things—name, address, phone, insurance, reason for the visit—to make it feel like I was receiving the proverbial 'third degree'. A fistful of papers, comparable to the stack at a real estate closing, had to be signed. By the time it was done, I was sure I'd signed away my first born, which seemed a real feat for someone not yet married. When my name was called, a courteous nurse ushered me into an examining room for the first of two interminable waits. There is the tendency among all patients everywhere to think that theirs is the most pressing problem of all.

My wife explains this with the observation, "No problem is minor if it is your own."

No better illustration of this comes to mind than a former colleague who suffered from tinnitus, a constant ringing in the ears. No doubt it is a nuisance, but in no way is it life threatening. To hear him describe it, though, one would think that the bane of tinnitus far exceeds every other human affliction: cancer, heart disease, and AIDS.

That we all think our problem is the most important helps explain why the waiting seems so endless. And, of course, the longer the wait, the more urgent the problem seems. I soon discovered that the one thing worse than sitting in a waiting room is sitting alone in an examining room. At least the waiting room has the outdated magazines, the other miserable broken wretches, and the television. The examining room has those dreadfully pallid walls that offer less than nothing to look at. So the attention turns to whatever diversion is available. First, my fingernails capture my attention. But, that does not last. Then, oh, to discover the intricacies of a jar of cotton swabs, or a blood pressure cuff. The mind, too, becomes its own burden. What will the doctor be like? Young? Old? Male? Female? Black? White? American?

"Please God," I silently prayed. "Let it be someone who speaks and understands English."

Self-doubt sets in. "I don't feel so bad sitting here like this. Do I really need to be here? I don't want to find out that it is one of those afflictions modern medicine can't cure. Let me die happy rather than discover something that will leave me a cripple for the rest of my life."

The curse of the mind ended the moment the doctor entered. Immediately, his youthful appearance struck me. I was brought up to think of doctors and policemen as my seniors. Before I had time to explore my doubts as to whether this child was competent to take care of me, the battery of questions begins.

"What brings you here? How long has it been going on? Do you have any family members with the same problem?" And on and on. Little did I know that the price of visiting a teaching hospital was volunteering for practice by medical students, interns, and residents.

It soon becomes apparent that the first doctor was not the neurologist. As I later learned, there is a medical specialty, 'emergency medicine', that deals specifically with patching up the 'walking wounded' who stagger into the Emergency Room. My youthful physician was probably an intern, a medical school graduate beginning his first year of specialization. This entails serving a year 'in the trenches' taking care of anything and everything that happens into the emergency room. A cursory examination reveals that I have 'brisk' reflexes, an indication of neurological involvement. Just what I don't want to hear.

"At least," I reassure myself, "I've come to the right place."

The adolescent with the stethoscope explains that a neurologist will be in to see me. If this haggard soul was unable to identify the problem, let alone fix it, at least he had the ability to recognize that I needed a neurologist.

Another interminable wait ensues while the intern searches for a neurologist. Meanwhile, I have more time to wonder. "What does it all mean?" Never having occasion to consider the nature of neurological illness, I begin to worry. Memories of an old college friend suddenly flood my mind. I recall the occasion when Bill mentioned something about having medical troubles in his brain, but never explained just what they were. Could he have had seizures? Something worse? All I know is that I don't want to mess with anything having to do with my brain. Heck, a broken bone, a torn ligament, appendicitis, anything but a problem with the 'main frame'. It isn't quite like a hangnail, and I want absolutely nothing to do with it. I was so intimidated by the idea of a problem involving my brain, I was afraid even to contemplate it. Would it be one of those things the movies portray where they can't decide whether or not to tell the patient? I could not help but wonder.

By now my sides were wet with perspiration. And I had not even been examined, let alone diagnosed. Heavens, at this point I was not convinced I wanted to be. The thought terrified me more than two decades ago, and I don't exactly warm up to it now.

A large black man entered. "Hello, I'm Dr. Durazel."

I didn't know whether to be relieved, or aghast. My worst fears had come true: this one had an accent! Soon enough I learned that Dr. Durazel was born in Haiti, fluent in English, and possessed a charming French accent. His calm demeanor and self-assurance quickly dashed all my doubts. In no time at all, I forgot his foreign birth and accent.

My fears about a foreign doctor reflect an unfortunate truth about many of us. We associate competence in speaking English with intelligence. Applied to native English speakers, this is not unreasonable. Regarding those raised speaking another language, however, it's nonsense. Two examples immediately come to mind. First, my grandmother, a Russian immigrant, lived in the United States ninety years without mastering the language. I distinctly remember the year she returned from her annual winter foray to Miami Beach, after the first great immigration of Cubans. Frustrated with the language barrier of a native Spanish-speaking hairdresser, she complained,

"I just can't understand why dem Cubans can't loin Hinglish!"

Not a person who knew her would suggest that my grandmother was anything but shrewd in every way.

To be sure, there is a legitimate concern that it might not be possible to communicate with one's physician. My experience with students who were not brought up speaking English has taught me otherwise. Those people who have had to learn English as a second language are more precise than those brought up speaking unaccented, bad English.

The story of an elderly acquaintance, my second example, illustrates the point equally well. Mr. Wolf, a retired letter carrier, was born in Transylvania, Romania. Despite living more than half his life in the United States, he still retained a pronounced accent. Many people had difficulty understanding his English. Nevertheless, he wrote the most lucid, well-argued, persuasive letters-to-the-editor published in the newspaper.

Still, the complaint persists, "But my physician can't understand me."

My answer is quite simple: let him or her tell you that. More often than not, a new language is understood before it is spoken. Every physician will tell you that one of the worst problems they face is the inability of patients to describe their symptoms accurately. In this regard, a neurologist I know teaches his students about the 'Neanderthal response'. To determine sensory levels, the point at which feeling still exists, he gently touches the skin with a sharp object. Attentive patients can describe where sensation drops off. Others will let out a loud grunt when the sharp object reaches an unaffected area, a 'Neanderthal response'.

A final point concerning foreign-born physicians bears explaining. Too many people mistakenly believe that foreign-trained physicians cannot be trusted. The American medical establishment shares this concern as well. Rest assured, they are every bit as competent as every other physician licensed in the United States.

The neurological exam Dr. Durazel performed was completely unfamiliar to me, but it should not have been. I had forgotten my visit to a neurologist when I was an undergraduate. But there was no reason to have remembered it. After all, I was in the prime of my immortality. On that occasion, I presented with a slightly numb left forearm and left thigh. The neurologist must have performed a modified exam, since he charted diminished sensory levels. Little did I know that that was the first foreshadowing of the MS to come ten years later. Dr. Durazel's pushing and pulling, pricking and tickling were both curious and mildly amusing.

Not knowing what it was all about helped me endure the investigation. Interestingly, just being touched by a physician seemed to make me feel better. Others have expressed similar feelings of being reassured by a physician's touch. Herein lies one of the secrets of chiropractors' success. Without taking anything away from the results they achieve, their manipulations have a substantial placebo effect because they convey a sense of actually fixing whatever is wrong. We can literally feel them fixing our problems.

Everything seemed to go swimmingly—who was I to know otherwise? Then, Dr. Durazel attempted to look at my optic nerves in the back of my eyes. He focused a beam of light into the eye with an ophthalmoscope, making is possible to look at the retina, or the butt end of the optic nerve. This unique 'open window into the nervous system' frequently reveals neurological problems. All this is contingent on the physician being able to focus on the retina. With those of us who are myopic (near sighted), this is problematic because we have elongated eyeballs. It wasn't until Dr. Durazel got on his hands and knees on top of me, as I lay on the examining table, that he was able to bring the backs of my eyes into focus.

"I do not think it is anything demyelinating," he assured me.

I acted reassured, which was easy because I had no idea what demyelinating meant. Neither did I have any idea how he could have concluded that any demyelination was occurring. Nevertheless, I heaved a sigh of relief.

Dr. Durazel continued, "We'll admit you for tests."

I didn't know what to say. I thought, "But you said it wasn't anything demyelinating. Doesn't that settle it?"

Rearing up in a combination of confusion of anger, resentment, and fear, I responded, "Not today you won't."

I promised to return three days later, on Monday.

Physicians are wonderful about these things. They act as if it is possible for all of us to interrupt our lives without notice, put all our affairs on hold, and follow their orders. Of course, in life threatening situations, following all orders immediately is essential. I concluded, however, in my infinite medical wisdom, no emergency was at hand.

With the doctor's words about it not being anything demyelinating—whatever that was—still ringing in my ears, I convinced myself that it was merely a muscle problem. I'd just have to work a little harder at exercising it out. Feeling rather buoyed by the whole experience, not to mention satisfied with my own diagnosis, I remained too stubborn to allow myself to learn anything from it. I proceeded to walk home—about two miles. True to form, my limp was worse than when I started.

What is the significance of presenting MS? For the longest time I was unable to answer this question. As an adolescent, I facilely dismissed it with all the hubris of youth. Sure, I had allergies, but so what? I'd blow my nose now and again. If a cat scratched me and I developed an itchy welt, I'd rub around it for relief. Sporadically I suffered backaches, but who didn't? I'd just tough 'em out. Little did I know that they were actually the early stages of ankylosing spondylitis, a potentially crippling form of arthritis. Even when diagnosed, I simply shrugged it off.

The true meaning of having a chronic illness still escaped me. The day my older daughter was prescribed eyeglasses drove the lesson home for me. When she was two and a half, her baby sitter reported that one of our daughter's eyes was looking at her nose. My wife recognized two possibilities: it could signal either an imbalance in the relative strength of her eye muscles, or a brain stem tumor. The latter is inoperable, and virtually fatal. Too nervous to hazard a diagnosis of her own daughter, we called our 70+ year old pediatrician, with more than forty years experience. We spent an extraordinarily restless night waiting. Recalling how his son developed the same condition at almost the same age, he didn't even bother to examine our daughter. He referred us to a pediatric ophthalmologist. We heaved a sigh of relief, dutifully took our daughter off to the ophthalmologist, and received a diagnosis of amblyopia (lazy eye) and far sightedness. For the former, he prescribed an eye patch for the stronger eye (and subsequently an operation on both eyes), while for the latter, eyeglasses.

What a revelation. Sure, she had suffered ear infections and an occasional cold, but they were passing maladies that affected an otherwise perfect child. Glasses represented a genuine imperfection. I was aghast at the thought. After all, hadn't I created a perfect child? My wife brought me back to reality.

"What are you getting upset for?" she asked. "Think of the alternative. At least she won't be dead."

Less than a moment's reflection left me humbled at my arrogance, and humiliated by my naiveté. From my daughter's need for eyeglasses, the true meaning of chronic illness finally occurred to me. Until that episode, I was still laboring under the misconceptions of youth.

The freedom of youth ends with the presentation of a chronic illness. From that time forward youth yields to maturity. No longer can we take our bodies for granted. We must learn to live with the imperfections, and disabilities illnesses impose against our will.

2

The Hospital

MS almost invariably includes time in the hospital. Whether the occasion is tests, routine treatment, or emergency measures, hospitalization can become commonplace. Among the hospital staff, we are referred to as either 'frequent flyers' or, as I prefer, 'repeat offenders'. Whichever way it is described, the result is the same. My calling MS sufferers 'repeat offenders' is based upon the similarity of hospitalization and incarceration. Once our i.d. bracelet is affixed, it is comparable to the handcuffs being slapped on a convict. When to sleep, when to get up, when to eat where to go, what to do, when we can visit with outsiders, and a whole myriad of other things are controlled by the authorities. Quite simply, we are no longer free. We can always leave the hospital 'AMA' (Against Medical Advice), but that is utterly foolish.

During a recent incarceration my roommate was ordered to bedrest, lest he jostle his cracked neck cartilage. If he did, the chief resident warned, he would likely end up a quadriplegic or dead. As my roommate was leaving, having ignored the pleading of friends, family, and a social worker, I mused with the chief resident,

"I bet he'll show up in the obituaries within two weeks."

Glumly, the chief resident agreed. I didn't have the heart to check the newspaper to see whether my prediction was correct. So much for leaving AMA.

Nothing about hospitalization recommends it aside from the prospect that we might leave in better shape than when we entered. I make the results of hospitalization conditional because there are so many aspects to it that can challenge the well being, physical, emotional, and psychological of even the healthiest individual. Because MS sufferers are often repeat offenders, it is helpful to begin with some advice that will improve the chances of leaving in better condition than when we were admitted.

It is better to swallow our pride, endure the indignities, and make the best of our stay in 'the joint'. Ever since my first hospitalization I refer to the hospital that way. I learned the term from the swimming pool attendant at a college where I taught for a year. He had served twenty-two years on death row for murder before being paroled.

Waiting

Nothing pervades hospital existence more than waiting. From waiting to be seen by the admissions office to waiting to be discharged, we seem always to be waiting for someone or something. Thus the first rule for a patient to learn is how to wait patiently, if not gracefully. (Is that where the use of the term 'patients' came from?) Short of that high expectation, at least we might be able to learn how to wait without completely losing our minds.

If this important lesson is not learned, the entire hospitalization will seem to blur into one interminable wait, punctuated only by occasional moments of generally disagreeable interruptions.

Unexpected delays are inevitable. Some likely causes are the following:

<u>Reason No. 1</u>: "The computer is down, I'll have to do this by hand." This generally will be followed by someone cursing that computer, all computers, or 'the stupid son-of-a-bitch who bought these damned things'. All we can do is smile, agree, and be glad we are not ten down on the list of people to be seen.

<u>Reason No. 2</u>: "An emergency came up." This can be any number of things, none of which is questionable. Whether it is a genuine medical emergency, the next patient showed up late, or a case of the person we are waiting to see has diarrhea, makes no difference. The bottom

line is, things have not remained on schedule, and we are not in a position to challenge it. The only option that will preserve our sanity, not to mention our blood pressure, is to sympathize, and remember all the emergencies that have ever thrown us off schedule.

Reason No. 3: "The last person took more time than expected." Medical treatment of every sort must be done well, not quickly. Before getting angry, we must consider what we would say to the next person in line if our case took longer than usual? How would we feel if we were given the 'bum's rush' just for the sake of staying on schedule?

Reason No. 4: "I have felt out of sorts since the moment I woke up today, and just can't get going." Typically, we refuse doctors the right to be out of sorts, if not outright sick. This reminds me of the unreasonable expectations children put on their parents. Under few, if any, circumstances do children understand, or accept their parents' problems or illnesses. This is understandable from children, but not from adults. If we are annoyed because of the wait it has caused, just remember how long the wait would have been if they had stayed home.

Reason No. 5: "Your doctor has been slow to respond because they have been working for the last 36 hours." No other profession expects practitioners to work continuously for that long. We should be delighted they showed up at all.

Reason No. 6: "They brought the person ahead of us down late." See Reason No. 2.

The natural human tendency is always to blame the messenger for bad news. We should be scrupulous to avoid this most common and human failing. We can complain all we want about the situation, but it should never be done in a way that gives the person listening the impression that he is the object of our dissatisfaction. Otherwise, we will assuredly learn a new meaning of the word wait.

Admission

Aside from those who are admitted on an emergency basis, and preferably unconscious at that, almost everyone else must go through the admitting office. The people working there have an unenviable job. Indeed, it is one that no person in his right mind ought to take. From the patient's vantage point, it is only an extraordinary individual who can survive the admitting process the first time without exasperation. MS sufferers have to undergo the admitting process multiple times, and thus ought to develop some tolerance for its tedium, and humiliation.

First, one must wait to be interrogated by the admitting person. For the attentive neophyte this contains an invaluable lesson always worth bearing in mind: as anxious or uncomfortable as you might be, you are not the only patient in the hospital. This is not an excuse for uncivil or negligent behavior. Rather, it is normal for a patient to behave as if he is the only patient in the hospital. Not surprisingly, he expects the staff to act accordingly. If you doubt the veracity of this observation, just ask any nurse.

The responsibility of the admitting person is primarily to look out for the hospital's interests. They must gather information necessary to establish our existence, thus allowing the staff to administer treatment. Our address, age, sex (as if they cannot tell by looking), next of kin, religion, and so forth are among the questions every patient is asked. Loosely translated, looking out for the hospital's interest means determining who is going to pay the bill. Patients are prone to resent this, but shouldn't. For A variety of reasons, an extraordinary number of patients cannot afford to pay. Meanwhile, the hospital still has to pay its overhead: staff, insurance, laundry, maintenance, and utilities, not to mention, new supplies and the latest equipment. This includes protecting the hospital's legal interests, as well.

The patient is asked to sign a host of releases: one for treatment, a second for the release of records, and on and on. In the end, we are certain that we'll need treatment for carpal tunnel syndrome in addition to whatever occasioned our visit in the first place.

Next, the admitting person presents us with a large envelope in which our valuables will be 'stored for safekeeping'.

Alas, our identification bracelet is affixed. And then, in the first act that demonstrates that our sentence has begun, we are told to sit in a wheelchair so someone can take us to our room. This has nothing to do with our condition, but reflects the hospital's legal responsibility for us. It fears that a lawsuit might ensue if we should fall on the way to our room.

A final note on the admitting person: if an admission is elective, it is possible to bypass the ordeal simply by pre-registering. Many hospitals allow patients to fill out the required forms ahead of time. Needless to say, this is always the preferable thing to do.

Our Room

The Hospital 'Johnny'

Even before we have time to take full account of the room, a nurse appears.

"Get into your pajamas," she orders. "If you don't have any, there is a gown on top of the pile of linens. I'll be back in a little while."

Here it is the middle of the day. We've been dressed since early morning. Now we are told to get into our pajamas! As one who relishes a midday nap, I will never forego the opportunity, but never in my pajamas. That is irrelevant in the hospital. Pajamas, we soon discover, are the official patient uniform.

If we knew enough to bring our own pajamas, an essential for every hospitalization, we are safe. But woe to him who must don the infamous hospital 'johnny'. One glance at it and we doubt the sanity of the nurse who referred it as a gown.

"Where's the back?" I wondered, holding up this smock by any other name.

The johnny is a mid-thigh length, wrap-around smock designed for the convenience of the medical practitioner. It facilitates easy examination of the patient. With nothing but a string tie at the top of the back, and another six inches below that to fasten the gown closed, one's buttocks is exposed for all to see.

Herein lies one of the great lessons of patient life in a hospital: there is no modesty. Doctors and nurses generally try their best, but the sad truth is that much of what they do leaves less than nothing to the imagination.

This lesson came home to me most poignantly the first time I invited the female neurology resident (now my wife), to join me for dinner. She performed the first extensive neurological examination on me after I was admitted. I didn't realize quite how extensive it had been. After inviting her, she paused a few seconds, and then continued,

"I don't know if I'll recognize you with your clothes on," she said.

Fortunately, the conversation transpired on the telephone. Otherwise, she would have seen me blush.

I have come to realize that regardless of what we might think of our body, the medical community regards it rather impersonally. 'Clinically', is the official term they use. In the same way an auto mechanic views an engine as out of tune, the hospital community views a patient as a human machine in need of repair. This is not entirely fair. We all know physicians and nurses who take a very personal interest in our welfare. My overstatement is intended to convey the notion that by viewing us clinically, the medical community can avoid the problem of becoming emotionally involved with us. Personal involvement can cloud one's judgment. It is for this reason that most physicians will not treat their own families for anything but the most minor illness. So, while we might be self-conscious about our most intimate parts, it is well to remember that to them, it's a body in need of assistance or repair. Besides, they've seen a thousand or more just like ours before.

Happily, there is a means by which even the johnny can be made to protect a shred of modesty. Wearing two of them, one facing frontward, the other backward, does the trick. This arrangement was shown to me by nurses who were sympathetic to the problem. Better still, forewarned is forearmed: bring your own pajamas. As one who has not worn conventional pajamas since childhood, I brought a silk-screened T-shirt, and boxer shorts. If I am admitted to the hospital on an emergency basis, I have someone bring them to me as soon as possible.

The Bed

Hospital beds are not made for sleeping. Two features about them convey this message. First, they make the firmest hotel bed feel soft and mushy by comparison. Merely sitting on them makes this abundantly clear. They do not yield beneath our weight. Sleeping on them is like a night camping without a pad beneath our sleeping bag.

The prison comparison becomes clearer by the minute: first, the shackle, next the humiliating uniform, and now this. What will be next?

The analogy soon breaks down when we realize the hospital bed has a particular corner on discomfort all its own: a rubber sheet on the mattress guaranteed to make us perspire profusely. As if it is not enough to make us sleep on the ground all night, it has to be a rainy night at that. Now the need for this little torture is unquestionable. Replacing soiled mattresses is far too expensive a burden for any hospital to bear. Regrettably, this logical and true explanation does nothing to make the rubber sheet any more comfy.

As with the imperfect-but-better-than-nothing-two-johnny solution to the modesty problem, there is a comparable solution to the tortuous bed. For the excessive firmness I ask for an 'egg crate'. This is a 1-inch thick, bed-sized pad of foam rubber, covered all over with rubber bumps that resemble an egg carton. Some hospitals have abandoned these because they tend to grow mold to which many patients are allergic. Alternatively, there is an air bladder. Neither is a panacea, but if we're stuck in the hospital, at least we won't feel as though we're sleeping on the naked ground. Regrettably, this does not entirely solve the discomfort of the rubber since the egg crate is foam, and the air bladder is covered with vinyl. Neither is a joy to sleep on. I suggest you request double sheets. Two layers of cotton are far better than one.

Hospital beds do have one distinct advantage. They allow us to raise, or lower our upper or lower torso at the touch of a button. Newcomers and children find this a great source of entertainment for around 10 minutes, the latter until they have been threatened to within an inch of their lives.

The Personal Patient Care Kit

One of the first items brought to us is a plastic-wrapped basin with all the goodies someone thought we might need to attend to our personal needs, washing, and grooming. What illegal substance the person who put these things together must have been smoking, one can only imagine. The items they contain are a rare combination of the ridiculous and irrelevant. Experience has taught me that there is slight variation in these kits from one hospital to the next. Nevertheless, every hospital charges for them handsomely.

A general description will suffice to convey their unique flavor. The most essential items are the wash basin, soap dish, water pitcher, and cup. So far so good, but there is also this mysterious kidney shaped dish made of the same plastic as the wash basin. Various people told me different things as to its proper use, brushing one's teeth, rinsing the mouth, but the one I found most implausible was as an emesis basin. Now, emesis is one of those wonderful medical words that has the salutary effect of making it possible to describe an unpleasant, but undeniable aspect of life, in a clinical way. At the same time, it makes doctors sound sophisticated, and patients stupid. Emesis derives from the Greek root emein, to throw off. That they choose not to call it what it is, baffles me. What is more incredible is the fantasy that any emesis, larger than a hamster's, could be contained by this dish. Regardless, they are useful for rinsing one's mouth after brushing the teeth.

This leads to another bit of essential advice: bring your own. The toothbrush included in the kit is too often more appropriate for scraping the paint off a battleship. Hard as I tried, I never succeeded in finding the 'rejected by the American Dental Association' stamp. They must have repackaged them. Don't forget the toothpaste. Kits are unpredictable, so it is impossible to know ahead of time whether there will be any in the one the hospital provides. Mouthwash tends to be another regular essential that regularly shows up. Heaven knows, bad breath is a ticket straight to Hell.

Other essential, but nearly useless personal grooming aids, are: a pocket comb like the kind adolescent boys carried in their back pocket in the1950's, a razor (but no shave cream) guaranteed to scrape enough skin off to make every pore gush with blood (pray they don't have to use it anywhere more intimate), an emery board, and an orange stick for cuticles. These call to mind the practice of scrubbing our homes spotless before leaving on vacation. On the one hand, this is logical for people who don't want to return to a messy house. On the other, there are those who worry that other people (friends, relatives, neighbors, police or fire departments) might have to enter their home, and could possibly find it messy. So with emery boards and orange sticks, for those whose deepest fear is that they might have to greet visitors with ragged cuticles. We should not become entirely skeptical. Hand and body creams are a staple that can be useful when receiving a soothing backrub.

The Food

Patients love to complain about hospital food. It tastes awful, is ill-prepared, cold, or any number of various criticisms. More often than not, these criticisms are unwarranted. The food begins as the highest quality available, and is prepared according to the most exacting standards. No hospital would risk a lawsuit by doing anything less. Prepared in enormous quantities, and restricted by the wide variety of medical demands, nutritionists and kitchen staff do remarkably well. This defense does not begin to account for the ridiculous variation in tastes the hospital kitchen is expected to satisfy.

With that much said, however, many patients can expect some unpleasant eventualities to follow from the typical hospital diet. Foremost among them is constipation. Although the Surgeon General has been stressing a high fiber/low fat diet, the message seems not to have reached the nutritionists. The one item that seemed most difficult to obtain on a regular basis is fiber. To be sure there is the bran cereal and prune juice option for breakfast, but after that getting adequate fiber can be a genuine challenge. Neither of the main course options for lunch or dinner will likely contain any fiber. Nor will the carbohydrate, for example, boiled white rice. The whole wheat bread is mostly white flour, and the vegetables are cooked until battleship gray. Regardless of their original color, anything cooked that long is sure to be unappetizing. The fresh salad is generally iceberg lettuce, cucumber slices, and a tomato wedge. No fiber. Alternatively, most uncooked vegetables come buried in Jello. The worst of both worlds. The fresh fruit option may be the best bet, but there is an even chance that it might be something with little or no fiber: a banana for example. On the other hand we might get lucky and get an apple or pear, both high fiber fruits.

To be fair, the low fiber diet along is not alone responsible for constipation. Spending most of the day in bed eliminates one of the great stimulants to regularity, physical activity. My own solution is ordering as much fruit as possible, asking friends and family to bring to whatever they can, and drinking as many hot liquids as I can tolerate. In contrast, it is possible to eat a diet so rich in fat that it would make a cardiologist cringe. Eggs for breakfast daily, meat or hard cheese at every meal, butter likewise, french fries on request, and cake or ice cream at lunch and dinner are staples of hospital diets. How naïve of me to think that hospitals would take the lead in insuring the good nutrition of their patients. Fortunately, it is possible to maintain a low fat diet by eating cereal at breakfast, substituting cottage cheese or yogurt for meat, and avoiding the rich desserts.

In fairness to the dietitians, the availability of all that fat is attributable to the desire to accommodate patients' desires. Patients feel miserable enough just being in the hospital, so everything possible should be done to make them comfortable. In keeping with this logic, patients should understand that the best way to get what we want is to ask for it. Food service will do everything possible to satisfy our wishes. I was on a course of steroid treatment that made me terrifically hungry. Regularly, I would order a midnight snack (or two) with my dinner. Without objection the food service would send me an extra sandwich or two with dinner.

The Roommate

Roommates come in all shapes, sizes, ages, and colors. They are assigned randomly according to the order of admission. Whoever we get, for good or ill, can only be attributed to coincidence. As this is the person with whom we are going to spend most of our time, the wisest course of action is to do the best to get along.

Never did I have to bear this in mind as much as on the occasion of my first hospitalization. A hospital neophyte, I was just settling into the strange new surroundings, when in walked two police officers, complete with service revolvers. Between them hobbled a man in shackles and leg irons. Nervous does not begin to describe how I felt. Madly, I searched my conscience to discover what I might have done to deserve this. Wasn't my curious limp and hospitalization enough? Nothing came to mind.

"This is Zachary," one of the officers told me. "He's come here to see what's wrong with his neck."

His neck looked fine to me. It was his leg that looked like it needed attention.

Although we were both single, and the same age, 30, all similarity ended there. He was black, I'm white. He was a Muslim, I'm Jewish. He was raised in the inner city, I'm a product of the suburbs. He didn't graduate from high school, I hold a Ph.D. He spent the previous 11 years in prison for murder, I was either in college, graduate school, or teaching as a professor. He wanted to be in the hospital, I didn't.

At this moment, we were identical in one crucial respect. We were both getting medical treatment. Our shared need for hospitalization, regardless of different reasons, obliterated even the widest differences between us. Wearing the same hospital Johnny, the richest and poorest are indistinguishable. My experience as an adolescent came to mind. At some insufferably early hour in the morning I would sometimes go fishing on the town pier. We were all convinced that the fish bit best at that most horrid time. On the pier everyone was equal. From the tax attorney, to old 'Portugee Joe, to an adolescent kid, we were all just fishermen waiting for dinner to bite. Lying in a hospital room with this stranger in the next bed, it made no difference who he was. We were both just patients.

My interest in Zachary was to learn something about human nature. I firmly believe that we can learn a lesson about life from every person. Some are worth emulating while others a are quite the opposite. To learn those lessons, however, we must first pay attention. Only the most arrogant among us believe they already know everything there is to be known about life.

The key to getting along with people is an interest in learning, even amid the artificiality of shared hospital incarceration. Of course, this is easier said than done. While we are tolerating the discomfort of illness, the hospital, or both is not an ideal circumstance. Learning about life through our roommates can fill the vacuum of time hospitalization creates. The most common activity otherwise is anticipating the next meal. Consuming it is regularly done at a breakneck pace. Ten or fifteen minutes later there is nothing left to do. Conversing with a roommate can at least distract from the pain of our own condition. Better than that, it holds out the promise of teaching us something about life.

So it was, for five days that I learned of a life full of potential, wasted on crime. Zachary turned out to be intelligent, as well as affable. His yarns about the crime that landed him in jail for life had little in common with the official record the guards shared with me. As he had immense amounts of time on his hands in prison, he had read extensively, though not wisely. I spent many hours trying, unsuccessfully I'm sure, to disabuse him of the conviction that there is a secret Jewish conspiracy to take over the world. He refused to entertain the idea that the <u>Protocols of the Elders of Zion</u> was proven to be a forgery. Likewise, he refused my entreaties that if there was such a conspiracy, I wanted my slice of the pie.

Zachary did not spend all his time chasing falsehood. Having become a competent chess player, he delighted in nothing so much as defeating me. The time I caught him off guard, and checkmated him earned his undying respect. That I was able to retain my composure despite having to share a room with a convicted murderer was attributable to two things. First, Zachary was not the first murderer I'd met. Second, there was a guard wearing a gun with us at all times.

My composure was challenged to the limit, however, the afternoon Zachary turned his amorous designs on me. Once he realized his advances toward the nurses, medical students, or anything else female were destined to go nowhere, I became the object of his desires. After repeatedly declaring in the most unambiguous terms that I am a very committed heterosexual, I took the first available opportunity to tell a guard.

With a stern expression, he assured me, "If he gives you any shit, I'll manacle him to the bed."

Thankfully, it never came to that, but I didn't sleep especially well the last two nights we shared a room.

There is an interesting story that can be told about each and every one of my hospital roommates. While none is as dramatic as my first 'trial by fire', each is memorable. That's just the point. The trials and tedium of hospital incarceration can be mitigated enormously by making a new acquaintance out of the poor wretch in the next bed. Maybe it's true, misery does love company.

One final note of caution: beware the roommate who says, 'Oops'. It indicates an incontinence problem, and signals the need to change the bed linens. During the day this is hardly bothersome, but several times per night has the potential to make a difficult situation considerably worse. There isn't much to be done about this, but in extreme circumstances it's not unheard of to request a room changes. Rest assured, however, if there is a solution, those responsible for changing all those linens will be the first to find it.

Staff

Residents

Residents are a fixture of teaching hospitals. Overworked and underpaid, these poor souls seem never to go home. As 'house staff' one of them has to be available at all times. Every third, fourth, or fifth night they are on call. They must be available to respond to the needs of all the patients being covered by an attending physician in their chosen specialty. Additionally, whenever an opinion (a consult) is requested in their specialty, they must respond. As a result, it is not uncommon for a resident work the entire night through. When they're on call, a 'work day' can begin at 7:30 A.M. one day, and conclude 36 hours later at 7:30 P.M the next.

Residents are apprentices in the fullest sense of the term. Fresh out of medical school, they are there to learn a specialty by practicing under the watchful eye of experts (attending physicians) in their chosen field. Unlike medical students, who pay the school so they can work ridiculously long hours, residents are paid apprentice wages—just enough for food and shelter. Calculated on an hourly basis, most make less than minimum wage.

There is a common misunderstanding that deserves to be addressed here. Many times people say about residents' long hours, "It's worth it, they'll make it all back later." Anyone who has seen the schedules residents keep, for the length of time required (3-12 years after 4 years of medical school), appreciates that money can hardly be their primary motivation. There are many easier ways for people with their intelligence and drive to get rich. To be sure, we all can name examples to the contrary, but they hardly disprove the general observation.

To a patient, residents are extremely important. Aside from the brief daily visit by the attending physician, they are our doctors. As medical school graduates and hospital employees, they are licensed to work as physicians. They write the daily orders of what is to be done, order tests, and prescribe medication. Although always under the watchful eye of an attending physician, the farther along they are in their training, the greater latitude they are given. It is not unusual for patients to see a resident more often than an attending, since a big part of their responsibility includes 'covering the floor'.

Consequently, a resident might well be more familiar with our particular case than the attending physician. Since their report is the basis for the attending physician's decisions as to which course of therapy to follow, their importance can hardly be overemphasized. Put simply, the resident can be our voice to the attending physician. If we can persuade the resident of something, chances are that the attending physician will order it for us.

As well, residents can overrule nurses. When a nurse insisted that I only needed to be catheterized once every four hours, I explained my dilemma to the resident. He understood my problem, and was sympathetic to it. He wrote an order in my chart specifying that I was to be catheterized whenever I requested it.

Occasionally, residents can be arrogant and condescending. Several years ago, I had a retired engineering professor as a roommate. In his sixty-something years he had never been hospitalized. Now, he was facing a cataract operation. Totally unfamiliar with hospital life, everything intimidated him. An ophthalmology resident stopped in, and I could hear him talking to my roommate as if to a child. The resident had to step outside the room for a moment. Meanwhile, I bristled. When he returned, I said emphatically, "I'm happy to see that you've met Dr. Schultz."

In no time at all, the resident's tone changed dramatically.

Residents can also be correct in judgment, while the attending physician can be wrong. On two important occasions this happened to me. The first was at a community health clinic when the resident correctly diagnosed my inflamed eye as iritis. An attending physician overruled him, and treated me for conjunctivitis. The second was during my first hospitalization when the resident thought I had MS, but the attending physician diagnosed me with another 'look alike', acute disseminated encephalomyelitis, a one-time illness. This latter was especially important since, in the intervening year between the misdiagnosis and the correct diagnosis, I married the resident who had been overruled.

Medical Students

If we are fortunate enough to be incarcerated in a teaching hospital, a score of medical students will take our history countless times. Every detail of our present condition, as well as every other condition our forbears ever suffered, will be recorded in copious detail. Learning to ask the relevant questions, and taking an accurate history are essential skills that every physician must learn. These fresh and enthusiastic doctors-to-be are not to be disdained. With considerably more time available than either attending physicians or residents, they are in the best position to answer questions. More than that, they can research our particular illness in the library, and be a source of valuable information.

As they know the hospital inside and out medical students are in a great position to get things done. Following a recent operation, I was transferred to the neurology service. The time to remove the stitches was long overdue. On her own initiative, a medical student spoke to someone in the neurosurgery department about it. Within hours a resident took the stitches out.

Nurses (RNs)

With the exception of our roommate, nurses are the people we see most often. As they are responsible for our minute-by-minute care, as well as conveying our needs to a physician, it makes overwhelming good sense to establish the best possible relationship with them. The rewards are well worth the modicum of effort it requires. Our requests are more likely to be addressed promptly and fully, not to mention pleasantly. There is no magic formula, or strict set of rules to be followed. The basic civility and decency that distinguish good character should not be abandoned once we become a patient. Nurses are skilled professionals, and deserve to be treated accordingly.

It may be easier to identify the characteristics of an undesirable patient than the reverse. With 5 to10 patients under their care, nurses have their work cut out for them. The last thing they need is a patient who demands to be treated as if he is the only one in the hospital. At any given moment there are likely to be two or more patients requesting attention. Whose call-light would we answer first? How would we determine who gets attention first?

Further, the patient who gives no indication of trying to get better is disheartening, as well as discouraging. The object is to be the patient they hate to see return to the hospital. Whenever I've made an encore appearance on the same floor, the nurses who know me greet me with a sorrowful, "What are you back here for?" Nurses want to see patients restored to full health probably almost as much as the patients do. This is especially true for those who have endeared themselves to them.

Nevertheless, there can be occasional moments of tension, no matter how hard one tries. During one stay, a middle-aged nurse and I crossed words over a minor disagreement. Individuals with MS suffer miserably from the heat. As the hospital seemed dreadfully hot to me one day, I removed my T-shirt. For no other reason than her own order, she asked me to put it back on. Much as I pressed the point, she would not yield. Dutifully, I put it back on until the shift changed. In the end it turned out to be a small price for maintaining the kind of relationship that resulted in attentive care.

More recently, there was a nurse who thought she knew more about the way my body behaves than I do. In most cases they do. As I am especially attentive to my body, I understand it rather well. Consequently, when it was time to go to physical therapy, I asked her to catheterize me.

She said, "It's too soon [since the last time]."

She refused to believe me, so I didn't press the point. I returned from physical therapy, prematurely, in need of washing and clean clothes. It's not that I went out of my way to prove her wrong, but she never balked at another of my requests to be cath'd.

Finally, patients frequently complain that they can never get a nurse when they want one. Allowing that there might be some truth in this, I have an utterly fail-safe method: go to sleep. In a split second a nurse will be there to rouse us. There is always a legitimate medical reason for these annoyances. Whether it is to take vital signs, give us a pill, or flush our i.v., a nurse well be there to prevent us from getting a good night's sleep.

Licensed Practical Nurses (LPN) and Nurse's Aids (NA)

In today's hospitals, LPNs and NAs do much of the work that used to be done by registered nurses. The financial climate necessitates saving money wherever possible. This explains why less highly trained nurses, and aids do as much as they do. This really makes little difference so long as the job is done well.

As these individuals are at the bottom of the medical hierarchy, they tend to have very little attitude about them. By the same token, they receive less training and are permitted to do fewer things. For example, they are not allowed to dispense any medication. Within the range of their responsibilities, however, both LPNs and NAs can be very competent and dedicated.

My experience with LPNs and NAs has been mostly positive. As long as they do their job well, honorably, and with pride, I respect them and treat them accordingly. This does not imply that I want to be their close friend, but only that I do not treat them disdainfully.

I am reminded of my secretary's position at work. Many of my colleagues feel that because they have advanced college degrees, that the secretary is an inferior human being...actually, a being of a different species might be more accurate. They fail to appreciate that their work would not be able to proceed without her. Rather than appreciate what she does, they act as if they have a divine right to her obeisance. At the hospital the phenomenon is comparable, but it is the LPNs and NAs at the bottom of the 'pecking order'. They deserve better.

Tests and Procedures

If the hospital uniform and the medical exam have not disabused us of all pretensions to modesty, the tests and procedures will. Guaranteed.

Tests are the essential scientific methods by which a physician's judgments are confirmed. We should take careful note here that these are not randomly selected tortures to be inflicted, but specific tools to 'rule out' various possibilities. Many illnesses can produce nearly identical symptoms. Each test adds another piece to the complex puzzle each illness presents. For example, an examination suggests that blood in the stool could be caused by: a simple bowel irritation, colitis, or worse, Crohn's disease. To determine which one, it may be necessary to subject us to the medieval torture of a colonoscopy. There are tests far worse, but few more undignified. The anticipation is always worse than the reality. With its ability to conjure up tortures not even medical science could imagine, the mind is far more sensitive than any other cells in our body.

Nevertheless, beware the words, "This may be a little bit uncomfortable." Doctors are masters of understatement. This calculated tendency is so as not to alarm the patient. Departure from this unwritten rule occurs only when a worrisome test has had positive results or a dangerous procedure or therapy has been a resounding success. At moments like these there is almost no end to exaggeration. Before a procedure, though, understatement has no bounds. The words 'a little bit uncomfortable' take on a whole new meaning. The best thing we can do is take heart and bear in mind, this, too, shall pass.

Some tests and procedures inevitably strip us of all modesty. When some stranger pokes into the most intimate parts of our anatomy, it is almost impossible not to be self-conscious. But, as with the johnny, the medical community sees little more than a body. When someone peers at a particularly intimate spot, we must remember that they are searching for evidence of disease. It only happens to be somewhere we'd rather keep to ourselves.

If many tests seem unnecessary, it is because medically they are. An enormous number of tests are performed as a matter of 'defensive medicine'. They are a physician's hedge against frivolous lawsuits. Decisions that used to be based on a practitioner's experience of thousands of nearly identical cases must now be grounded in the undeniable proof of tests. Judgment must take a back seat to the hard evidence of reproducible tests because every patient is a potential lawsuit.

Summary

The hospital is what we make of it. None of us enjoys being there, but too often that is not a choice we get. Knowing what is in store for us can make the entire enterprise more bearable.

Hospital staff is likely to treat patients whom they are particularly fond of especially well. This is not to say that everyone doesn't get perfectly decent, adequate treatment. But some patients get their call light answered a little faster, their food served a bit sooner, their requests honored a trifle more completely. Besides, if nothing else, these things are not done grudgingly. Hard as it is to believe, we must realize that we are not the most important patient in the hospital. Being arrogant, overbearing, or demanding is likely to have the opposite effect from what was intended. Instead of faster, more attentive care, we are likely to get resentful, precise care.

A patient is rendered likable with the same characteristics that make a desirable neighbor or friend. Affability goes a long way. Everyone knows the hospital is a miserable place to be, but acting miserably only serves to make us undesirable to be around. Asking for something frequently results in no one wanting to be close enough to listen. We can't expect to be treated like a prince (or princess) if we act like a boor. Being the patient everyone wants to hug when we are discharged, as well as the one everyone feels sorry to see when we are admitted, is the patient I try to be. It takes hardly any effort, and makes everyone's life considerably more pleasant.

3

Diagnosis: Now That You Have It, What Are You Going To Do With It?

Being diagnosed with a chronic illness can be harrowing. It need not be. My 'day of judgment' was actually two days of judgment. First, when I was diagnosed with ankylosing spondylitis. And then, with multiple sclerosis.

My different reactions to these two are instructive as a study in contrasts, neither of which I recommend. Beginning in my late teens, I had backaches. Sporadically, my lower back would become painful, resulting in a marked limp, always making me uncomfortable. I assumed the problem was muscular. That was the only source of discomfort I knew. I visited orthopedic surgeons. One after another they ordered x-rays of my spine, told me my bones were straight, and prescribed a variety of exercises. I diligently followed their orders, but the backaches persisted. At age 29, a painful red eye sent me to an ophthalmologist. After a brief examination he diagnosed iritis, a symptomatic diagnosis of an inflamed iris. In and of itself, that would have neither distressed nor impressed me. Then he stunned me with a question.

"Do you have lower backaches?"

When I affirmed that I did, he explained that there is an established correlation in young men between iritis and lower backaches. Before I could contemplate the meaning of it all, he continued.

"I'll send you upstairs [to a rheumatologist] for films."

Within minutes, my lower back was x-rayed. Upon a return visit the rheumatologist informed me that the x-rays revealed the possibility of ankylosing spondylitis [arthritis of the non-moving joint where the spine and pelvis meet].

He presented me with a prescription for six months of a non-steroidal anti-inflammatory medication. Since he never explained why I should continue taking it, I discontinued the medication a few days later once the pain disappeared. A few years later, I learned from my wife that the object of anti-inflammatory medication is to keep the swelling down, which prevents the pain from ever recurring.

I was not moved by the diagnosis. That was a combination of ignorance and arrogance. I neither knew what ankylosing spondylitis was, nor anyone suffering from it. That being the case, I had no interest in learning more about it. Whether I knew a great deal or not probably would have made little difference. Knowing more about the nature of nonsteroidal anti-inflammatory drugs would likely have spared me the discomfort of future bouts of lower back pain. To be fair, the fault belonged as much with the physician as with me, because he never explained that ankylosing spondylitis could cripple me.

My arrogance was nothing other than blithe disinterest in the nature and implications of my condition. It never even occurred to me to learn about it. After all, why should I? Being otherwise healthy, there was no reason to want to find out about an illness that had yet to become very serious. You see, I did not yet realize that I was not invincible. My feelings were typical folly of youth.

Being diagnosed with multiple sclerosis was completely different. It was an illness whose name I had heard, but nothing more. Exactly what it is, how it operates, what prospects it holds, and so forth were all foreign to me. I only knew that it was really serious, and I wanted nothing to do with it.

During my first hospitalization, MS was on the differential of possible diagnoses. When the available evidence seemed to point away from MS, a sense of relief that swept over the room. Everyone present, attending physician, resident, and medical students heaved a collective sigh of relief. So did I, without fully knowing why. My neurologist concluded that it was acute disseminated encephalomyelitis (ADEM). Its name was irrelevant to me. All that mattered was that unlike MS, it would go away. Only later did I learn that 20% of ADEM sufferers die. With the knowledge that ADEM wasn't chronic, I felt free to pursue my life with no changes, except for the time off from work that recovery demanded.

Nine months later I was married, not giving the prospect of chronic illness a second thought. Six weeks into my marriage, my wife noticed me slurring my speech. She knew immediately what it meant, although she didn't tell me. For my part, I was unaware that anything was amiss. Shortly thereafter, we were invited to a dinner party where my neurologist was also invited. He noticed me slurring my words, and told me he wanted to see me in his office.

During that office visit he told me that it was MS. It was as if the jury had just come in, pronounced me guilty, and sentenced me to death. I was devastated. A million emotions swirled through my head at once. Will I get worse? In which ways? When? Will I be a cripple? What will become of my marriage? Can I father children? If so, what kind of father will I be? I remembered how my mother died when I was 12 years old. Do I want children, if their father is going to die at a young age? Then, of course, it struck me. How soon would I die? I was reminded of a joke. Question: what do you want people to say at your funeral? Answer: he sure was old. I heard the diagnosis, but because my life was largely unaffected, I did everything in my power to deny it.

Denial is very common among people diagnosed with MS. Subsequent conversations with MS sufferers confirm this observation. Almost invariably, they will do almost anything to escape the prospect that may await them. It is not unusual for newly diagnosed MS sufferers not to want to meet with me. Fear of the future? Perhaps. Meanwhile, my own denial surged ahead full steam.

"Maybe he's finding things that aren't really there," I reasoned.

In retrospect my doubts were a form of avoidance. That was perfectly logical. Who would choose to have a horrific illness? Determined to prove my neurologist incorrect, I measured my body's every movement, always searching for confirmation that I didn't have MS.

Whenever my body responded well, I said, "See, I'm not truly sick. He was wrong."

The difficult times I conveniently ignored.

Another common reaction is an intense conviction to find the solution that nobody has found before. Understandably shocked by the bad news, people ask a million questions, doubt whatever diagnosis they were given, and research the disease themselves. That others have already covered the same ground is of little consequence. They want confirmation of their own. I know, I did.

My newly found confidence was short-lived. At home my emotions overcame me. I lay beside my wife, and cried like a baby as she held me.

As the tears poured down my face, I sobbed, "But I always wanted to be a grandfather."

In her pricelessly gentle, but totally disarming way, she reminded me,

"First, dear, you have to be a father."

Logic and rationality were wasted on me. I was grieving for my own future and didn't want to be interrupted. In a wave of self pity, I continued.

"Yes, but why me? Why now? What did I do to deserve this?"

Accustomed to seeing terminally ill infants, my wife responded,

"What do you mean? Why you? Why now? What about those newborns who are destined to die in two weeks, or two months from some agonizingly painful condition? What did they do to deserve it? You've had thirty good years."

She didn't have to remind me that in my thirty good years there were far too many reasons why I should contract this miserable illness, or worse. Unable to explain myself, I searched in vain for another explanation for the illness. My crying turned to cursing. Everything was fair game for my foul mouth. From the maker of the universe, to the capriciousness of my contracting the illness, nothing escaped my wrath. I was frustrated because no one could explain why I got MS, what its progress was likely to be, or what effects it would have on me. I was indignant because I felt that I deserved an explanation.

Sad to say, MS has none. Worrying about its cause is comparable to fretting over the reason for any disaster. Why do insurance companies call them "acts of God?" They have no logical explanation. Even being able to explain why MS happens, would change nothing. Not surprisingly, neither my crying, cursing, frustration, or righteous indignation changed anything, either.

Once the tears stopped, the cursing ceased, the frustration subsided, and the indignation receded, I was every bit as sick as before. All my carrying-on accomplished nothing, except exercising my lungs and wringing my tear ducts dry. My MS was completely unchanged. Like getting drunk or taking recreational drugs, the effects don't last. It is simply an exercise in futility. Worse, it wastes valuable energy needlessly and uselessly.

When I composed myself again, I thought I owed it to my family know of my diagnosis. By the time I called my older brother, I realized that I didn't have to be afraid to buy green bananas. Upon telling him that I was diagnosed with MS, he revealed his ignorance.

"How long have you got?" he asked.

I couldn't resist.

"'bout two weeks," I responded.

There was a long pause at the other end of the phone. I realized he had no reason to know about MS, so I told him the truth. Even now, I still have no answers to the whole myriad of cosmic questions. Nobody does.

Once my speech cleared up, my denial resumed. I continued searching for evidence that I didn't have MS. Every time I did something well, I took it as a sign that I was not sick. At the same time, I regularly overlooked all indications to the contrary. That I would drag my right leg most of a half mile to the swimming pool meant nothing, compared to my ability to walk home briskly following a half hour in an unheated pool. Just when I was almost convinced I really didn't have it, my feet began feeling too large for my shoes, my fingers became numb, and tingly, as if they were being crushed in a vise. I was having an MS exacerbation. My days of denial were over.

"Oh no, I really do have it," I lamented. "Now what?"

Two options presented themselves. First, I could define my life by the illness. A young woman at the college library illustrates this well. Right after being diagnosed, she bought a wheelchair, got in it, and spent her waking life therein. She simply consigned her life to the illness. Although I knew of her existence, I made it a point never to make her acquaintance. Her behavior seemed despicable to me. Defining my life by the illness is something I never considered doing and have never done. I take the Popeye view of life, "I yam what I yam, and that's all that I yam."

Second, I could define my life by the things I want to be. This is what I attempt to do. Regardless of anything else, according to all common definitions, I am a cripple. That neither troubles nor offends me, for I refuse to allow MS to define me. I do not want people to think "cripple" when they think of me. Consequently, I keep trying to march forward with the same goals I've always had, modifying them only as necessity dictates. Whether it is as a husband, father, teacher, or friend, those are the things I've always wanted to be. That MS has meant that I cannot do them as well as I would like is distressing, but it has not dissuaded me from aspiring to them. I readily admit, however, that I could be better in a zillion ways.

MS fundamentally attacks my body. In short, it makes life miserable. Happily, humanity has the unique ability to define life in other ways. Consider, for example, a newspaper obituary. How often do they describe someone according to their physical prowess or attributes? No, people are remembered by the distinctly human qualities they manifest. That is certainly how I want to be remembered. MS has not robbed me of them yet. I don't expect it ever will. I will never be allow to do that.

How we react to the diagnosis of MS is just one chapter in a lifetime of challenges. Indeed, it marks the beginning of a new life. Whether it will be for good, or ill is in our hands.

4

M.D. Does Not Stand For Minor Deity

Nowhere are the limits of modern medicine more manifest than in the treatment of multiple sclerosis. Since, by definition, it is destined not to be cured, the best that we can expect is that it be managed well. 'Managed' is the euphemism for 'kept down to a dull roar'. In practical terms this means that the symptomatic treatment is sufficient to make life bearable. While this is a source of frustration to many—they can put a man on the moon, but they can't even stop the ringing in my ears—it may be the best that today's medical knowledge can offer. Unless we accept this unpleasant reality, life will be a continual search for a magical physician with a miracle cure. If the limits of modern medicine are accepted, however, we will be able to develop realistic expectations and pursue reasonable judgment concerning the management of our illness.

The importance of having the right physician cannot be overstated. Our medical care, which controls everything from the quality of existence to our very life, depends on the practitioner we select. This begs the question, who is the best physician for me? Answering this question requires making certain calculations.

First, the quality of a physician is as much a function of the quality of the patient, as it is of the training of the practitioner. So, if we want the best medical care, it is essential that we be the best patient. How do we do that? It begins with a sober understanding of what we can reasonably expect from a physician. Typically, we expect too much. A student of mine, whose husband was a medical resident, joked with me once that 'M.D. does not stand for minor deity'. It would be funnier if it were not so close to the truth.

There is an old joke in the medical community. A major disaster occurred in which hundreds of people were killed. As they waited in line to pass through the pearly gates, a short, bearded man wearing a white lab coat, carrying a small black bag, and dangling a stethoscope from his neck scurried directly into heaven. After safely passing through the pearly gates, one inquisitive individual turned back to St. Peter, and asked, 'Who was that little man who ran past me?' St. Peter replied, 'Oh, that was God. Sometimes he likes to play doctor'.

Sadly, too many of us act as if this is what we believe. If there is something wrong, physicians must be able to diagnose, and treat it. More than that, we demand that they do so immediately, precisely, the first time, and preferably painlessly. For good measure they should also be able to accomplish this minor miracle for the same $8 a general practitioner charged in 1958. We forget that the general practitioner of the past could not begin to do what today's specialist can.

What makes us so nostalgic about the physicians of the past? In some measure they were able to inspire confidence. That they could not do a fraction of what today's practitioner can do is irrelevant. We believed in them because they genuinely cared about us. Is there any better explanation for the nostalgia over home visits? We fail to appreciate that the little black bag a physician carried had nothing magical in it.

Today, our anger is also partly attributable to our resentment of the salary doctors make. We are convinced that the only moving force in them is a lust for money. The gross statistics, however, are misleading. The average salary of a surgeon far exceeds that of an internist or pediatrician. Yet the statistics bandied about rarely make those distinctions. Instead, we prefer hating all 'rich doctors'. Mark Twain had it right when he said, 'There are lies, damned lies, and there are statistics'. To be sure, every barrel has some bad apples in it. By contrast, numerous doctors give away their services for free. That we don't bristle over the salaries of entertainers or athletes is ironic. They make as much in a single season as a physician (or almost any other professional) can in a lifetime. Yet, neither entertainers nor athletes have anything to do with our health or well being.

We are the victims of our own inflated expectations. If the doctor finds an illness, there must be a pill or potion to cure it. We assume it will be cleared up within a day or two, and the prescription will cost only a few dollars. How disappointed we are upon discovering that there is no 'magic cure', that we will simply have to endure whatever it is that ails us.

Sadly, I found myself guilty of this recently in the treatment of arthritis. Hoping to find something newer and better than my usual standby, I inquired of a physician-friend which medication he prescribes for arthritis these days. Much to my disappointment, he allowed that while there are probably thirty prescriptions on the market, none stands out from the rest. In fact, he explained, they all do about the same thing. The only challenge is to discover which gives us the most relief, and has the fewest side effects. Just what I didn't want to hear: no magic pill. Phooey! I would rather hear that a new medication had just been marketed, offered complete relief, had no side effects, and cost a pittance.

All of this indicates the importance of appreciating the limits of modern medicine. There are some illnesses and conditions which medical science cannot explain, let alone cure. That physicians understand those limits is evinced by their own reluctance to seek medical help for the conditions they suffer. Time and again, I've seen physicians who will neglect their own conditions, rather than seek medical help. It is a perfect case of the shoemaker's children going barefoot. Moving heaven and earth is easier than getting a physician to the doctor. Perhaps they appreciate how little medicine can actually cure. Equally plausible, they may be reflecting society's attitude concerning the omnipotence of physicians. For people who have spent more than four years learning to how to heal patients' maladies, and have had people telling them they are all-knowing, discovering that they are not omniscient and omnipotent is a very bitter pill.

Early in my marriage, I used to tease my wife that there must to be a course in medical school which teaches the students that the words, "I don't know", doesn't exist. Blaming medicine for this limitation changes nothing. Unpleasant as it is, we have no choice but to accept it. If we don't, we are likely to spend our lives being frustrated and bitter. Sad to say, such individuals really exist. They lead utterly miserable lives. It is arguable whose lives they make more unpleasant, their own or everyone around them.

Granting medicine's limits changes our calculus in finding a physician. Successful medical treatment of MS involves the combined efforts of doctor and patient. The best physician is the one who will make the best patient of us. Doing that begins with the physician being as much an educator as a medical practitioner. Patients need to be taught about their illness, and what relief medicine has to offer. My own experience with ankylosing spondylitis is an example of a physician's failure to educate the patient. I was never told that the object of an anti-inflammatory drug is to keep the pain of swelling from ever occurring. Hence, I was supposed to continue taking it, despite there being no pain. Similarly, consider how many times we have been prescribed 10 days of an antibiotic, told to finish the entire bottle, but never told why. My wife explained that the weaker germs are eliminated with the first few days of taking an antibiotic, but the stronger ones can endure. They require the full 10 days of treatment to be eliminated. So, now you know.

The greatest obstacle to physician education of patients is the cost. Talking to patients takes time, and time is all that most physicians have to sell. There is scarce remuneration for that. Regrettably, thinking and talking are not compensated at the same rate as performing tests and procedures. This is a reflection of our belief in science. We trust things if they can be 'proven' scientifically. Patients need to remember that a physician's practice bears all the burdens of any other business. All of the overhead expenses, from the cost of the office, to malpractice insurance, and the salaries of the employees, must be met. Nevertheless, the best physician realizes that time spent informing patients about their illness and its treatment are investments in keeping chronically ill patients 'well'. Additionally, education can keep patients from making unnecessary calls and visits to the office.

An equally estimable obstacle is physicians' lack of training as educators. They are trained in treating illnesses. Properly educating patients requires assessing the ability of the 'student' to be educated, knowing what information needs to be conveyed, as well as understanding how best to convey it. That a physician might be deficient in this regard is hardly surprising. Alternative sources of education are readily available to patients. Pamphlets detailing everything from the etiology (origin) of an illness to its treatment and prognosis are in every physician's office. Likewise, there is a web page detailing the origin and treatment of every conceivable illness on the Internet. Moreover, for those individuals more comfortable with verbal explanations, several national MS organizations are prepared to offer comfort, guidance, and assistance. Even the busiest doctor should be able to provide literature or direct a patient to the appropriate support group. It is clearly in their interest to do so.

The best physician will inspire our confidence. So much of the management of MS is subjective. As it cannot be cured, the quality of its management increases in importance. How we perceive the quality of the care we receive becomes an independent variable all its own. How many times have we heard, 'I'm going to Dr.—, he's one of the best in the country'. It is not very likely that he is one of the best in the country, although it is not impossible. More important, however, is how we perceive a physician's ability and the confidence it inspires. That we believe a physician is providing the best that medicine has to offer is crucial. If we believe this, then we are more willing to accept the reality of the limits of modern medicine. Equally important, we are more likely to follow the directives of our physician. Many pharmaceutical houses are actively engaged in producing medication that requires less frequent administration, ideally, once or twice daily. Patients can be trusted taking two pills daily rather than twice that number. Equally important, if we are going to be accountable to someone whom we trust, we are considerably more likely to be diligent in following instructions.

What do we look for if 'one of the best in the country' happens not to be nearby? A physician who conveys a sense of concern and caring for our well-being will inspire the confidence every patient needs and deserves. I have seen instances of physicians to whom I would be reluctant to take my pet guinea pig, yet I hear people rave about them. That our opinions can be so radically different is attributable to our different perceptions of the same practitioner. It is entirely possible that the patients in question genuinely believe that their physicians care very deeply and can genuinely help them. That alone is half the battle.

The best physician will enlist us as partners in the fight against the illness. We will be expected to follow instructions explicitly, and report any and all developments promptly and precisely. The finest physician will not be threatened by a patient's knowledge. Rather he or she will use it in conjunction with the latest medical technology to provide the best medicine has to offer.

If the best medical treatment depends on the best patient, what does it take to become the best patient? First, the best patient will want to get better. One of the rewards of being a pediatrician, I am told, is that the patients really want to get better. Such is not necessarily the case with adults. With MS, this is especially vexing because there really is no 'getting better' in the fullest sense of the term. Rather, there is only living as well as possible within the limits set by the condition.

Wanting to get better and being prepared to do everything in our power to that end is essential. The 'everything' in this case is fundamentally a disposition, not necessarily an activity like physical therapy. For whatever reason, too many of us do not want to shed the burdens of illness. Either we refuse to accept the reality of the MS or the limits of its treatment. A physician cannot make us better. We need to be a full, active participant in making our lives as full and rich as possible.

Second, more than simply wanting to get better, the best patient will do everything he can to relieve the condition. This is all relative, of course, because MS patients cannot get entirely better. Nonetheless, insofar as we are able to make our lives more bearable, it is incumbent upon us to do everything in our power toward that end. This includes physical as well as intellectual activity. Learning about our illness, in many respects, is as important as physically attempting to improve our condition. If we know what to expect and how to react to changes in our condition, then we will be better prepared for whatever our illness brings.

Above all, we must realize that no physician can make us better. At best he can relieve our condition and bring the latest developments of medical science to bear. That may not be a great deal, but an outstanding physician will make us realize that he is doing everything possible to relieve our condition. Beginning by realizing that he is not a minor deity is an important first step in forging a partnership against MS.

5

The Challenges of MS

Multiple sclerosis presents a variety of challenges. How we react to them can make the difference between a fulfilling and happy life, or a miserable and frustrated one. The choice, is in our own hands.

MS brought my life as I knew it to an end. Old goals were tailored to a bygone era. They suited a situation that no longer exists. Since MS changes the 'rules of the game', new goals had to be developed. The first challenge for me was figuring out just what the new rules are governing my life. That I had no hand in choosing or setting them made no difference. The reality was that I would have to live by them.

Even before addressing the dilemma of figuring out the new rules that govern life, I had to accept the reality of the illness. It began by realizing that my life is no longer my own. Indeed, it never will be again. Liking the illness is not an option. My feelings are irrelevant. Now, I must accept the reality that, willy-nilly, my life is shared with some dreadful illness. Worse than that, the illness has relegated me to the status of junior partner. It has the final say. I must begin with the premise that it is bigger, stronger, and tougher than I am. Overpowering it, or denying its existence is impossible at best, self-destructive at worst. I recall vividly how my brother reacted to the news of my diagnosis by recounting his response to a bout of bursitis.

"I just took the pills the doctor prescribed," he said defiantly, "and flushed them down the toilet."

Fortunately, the bursitis subsided, despite his foolish arrogance. Although I had no pills to flush down the toilet, I never considered that a sensible option. No, I realized that living begins by acknowledging that life's limits are established by an unwanted, if unavoidable, and inescapable master.

Acceptance has allowed me to think beyond the illness. Until then, hating everything in sight and fighting the illness were my major pre-occupation. Cursing and crying were the only two things I could do until I accepted the grim reality. Psychologists describe this common response as grieving. Would that it made a difference. Regrettably, it doesn't.

Once accepted, the illness became just another challenge for me to meet. There having been many in my life, I took it for granted that swimming upstream is what I should do. My mother's death when I was 12, 'mothering' my father and two younger sisters at 14, and leaving home at 19 to put myself through college, were all good preparations for this new challenge. Unlike the previous episodes, where I knew what had to be done, however, MS was different. It cast the future in doubt. Discerning what needed to be done became my responsibility. Little did I know that it would become a regular activity, and major preoccupation.

Every minute of every day I am reminded of MS is present. Whatever I do, wherever I go, it's with me. From the moment I awake and strain to get out of bed in the morning, until I struggle to climb into bed at night, I am never allowed to forget that I am carrying an additional burden. In thousands of ways perceptible to no one but me, I am constantly reminded of my illness. No matter how hard I try, there is no escape.

MS is just that insidious. It is a jealous master always demanding primary attention. When it says rest, I must rest. When it produces pain, relief is primary. There is no alternative. It can neither be ignored, nor scoffed. Woe unto the one who does either. Like it or not, the illness is the senior partner. I recall the last time I had a toothache. Nothing else mattered until that tooth was paid some attention. How absurd, not to say frustrating, that all of life had to be put on hold over one tooth. Yet whenever that happens, there is nothing we can do about it. MS is a toothache writ large. But unlike a toothache, MS is constant, relentless, and permanent. It demands more than attention. Obeisance more closely describes it.

Luckily, there has never been a tyranny so thoroughgoing and complete in the history of mankind that it has obliterated the human desire for freedom. The 20th century was witness to two of the most oppressive dictatorships ever known. Neither Nazi Germany nor the Soviet Union was able to suppress their citizens' yearning for freedom. So too with MS. It dominates and controls my body. Over that, I have no choice, but to compromise with it. Beyond that, however, my life is my own.

Discerning the limits the illness sets is a process of experimentation. Arguably, it is one of the most demanding and relentless of the challenges MS presents. By paying attention to my body's reactions to various conditions, the limits the illness establishes become manifest. From what I can do, how often, and for how long, to what I can eat or what I should avoid are all areas of exploration. Only in this way is it possible to find out the limits the illness sets. Do I ever go over the line and overheat or exhaust myself? More often than I care to admit. Sometimes I do so intentionally, knowing the price I will have to pay. Eating sizable quantities of carbohydrates, for example, especially the long chain varieties such as bread, potatoes, or pasta, raise the body temperature because they require more energy to be digested. I can count on them making me weak. Sometimes I eat them anyway. Knowing the full extent of what I can do is a constant process of testing the limits.

To complicate matters, the demands of my chronic illness are rarely stagnant. This is doubly true of a progressive, degenerative disease like MS. Unlike, say, a broken spine that permanently paralyses parts of the body, the disabilities and burdens of MS fluctuate. Depending on a myriad of conditions—physical, environmental, emotional, and psychological—the demands of the illness vary. Thus it is not enough that I have to pay tribute to an unwanted master; it is a master with changing demands. It's like pursuing a criminal who constantly changes disguises.

Frequently, people ask me whether I have better and worse days.

"No," I answer. "There are better and worse hours."

At different times of day and different atmospheric conditions, I know I will be affected in distinct, predictable ways. MS tends to be especially sensitive to the heat and humidity. There is an inverse relationship between my body's temperature and its ability to function. As the normal Circadian rhythms cause the body's temperature to rise in the late afternoon, I am at maximum weakness. Regardless of everything else, this is late day 'down time', or DT as we call it around my house. It is as predictable as the sun rising in the east. From around 4 o'clock until 7 o'clock, I am physically unable to do almost anything. Frequently, I am rendered so weak that I cannot lift a fork to my mouth. Two or three hours later, my body is back to baseline again, and I have trouble understanding why it was so difficult to do anything earlier.

Unusual rises in my body's temperature produce more serious effects. Around 15 years ago I contracted a virus that gave me a slight fever. As lay in bed, I discovered that my legs were paralyzed. I was concerned that the condition might be permanent.

I asked my wife, "Will it get better?"

"I don't know," she told me.

Never one to be daunted, she made me take an ibuprofen for the fever. In less than an hour I walked into the kitchen.

From this episode I learned the lesson of patience and determination. Patience is a particularly difficult idea for Americans to accept. My dissertation adviser taught me this.

"What's the most common word in advertising?" he would ask.

Answer, "New."

We are driven by the desire for the newest of the new, assuming that it will always be better. How long does the public pay attention to any single news story? MS does not take kindly to impatient patients. Neither does it react favorably to bullies.

A extreme example occurred in November 1994. Again, I contracted a minor virus, and my body reacted to the fever by going almost totally spastic [rigid]. When my neurologist stopped by, he found me sprawled on the floor, having failed in my attempt to walk into the bathroom. Regardless of how hard he tried, my body refused to bend. He concluded that it was better to allow the hospital to look after me. When I was admitted (7:30 P.M.) my temperature was 37.7 degrees centigrade [normal is 37.0 degrees]. The fever gave me the chills. Four hours later, I lay in bed (my temperature was 38.8 degrees) too weak even to push the call button for a nurse. I was completely quadriplegic. I was positively terrified. Three hours later, the fever broke. I awoke sweating. A day and a half later, I was discharged with my body back to 'normal'.

Thankfully, most of my time is not consumed with extraordinary problems. For regular weakness bred of the heat, I discovered that ice water or a popsicle temporarily restores my strength. In fact anything cold will have the same effect. Conversely, I find that the most effective way to warm myself up is from the inside out: drinking a hot beverage or eating hot food. A better solution is simply to avoid getting hot. So, I gave up wearing suit coats to work. Next to be abandoned were the T-shirts. Third to go were the neckties. Last, were the long sleeves. Today, I do not even own a long sleeve shirt. Both at home and in the office the thermostat is set in the low 60s.

Summer is the bane of my existence. Weeks will pass before I venture out of the air conditioning. It is not my first choice among desired lifestyles. I used to play tennis in the noonday Maryland sun, but it is the environment in which my body functions best.

People ask me, "Aren't you freezing?"

"Yes," I answer, "but I function better this way."

No longer am I self-conscious about not wearing a coat and tie in a room full of men wearing them. My need is to remain cool. If someone doesn't appreciate my manner of dress, that's their problem.

However constant the illness is, it can be unpredictable as well. New symptoms only confuse life further. Change, and adapting to it, is a constant in my life. Bladder problems are a case in point.

When I was first diagnosed, I learned that a sizable proportion of all MS sufferers experiences what physicians call 'retention'. Demyelinated nerves fail to conduct the signal to the brain that the bladder is not entirely empty. Hence, the bladder will give the impression that it is empty, when in fact it is not. Two possibilities can result from this condition: bladder infections and/or the need to urinate frequently. The surest solution is catheterization, because it empties the bladder entirely. I determined that I would not be one of those who experiences retention. There is no way on God's green earth that I will stick most of a 16" pencil-sized, rubber hose up my you-know-what. No way, not me, uh-uh! Tough talk.

Only a few years after being diagnosed, I found that the one-hour drive to school more than my bladder could take. Either I would have to stop along the way, or race for a restroom as soon as I arrived. Desperate for relief, I called my neurologist. He immediately diagnosed a small, spastic bladder and prescribed a muscle relaxer. Both my wife and I had our doubts. She suspected the opposite, a large flaccid bladder, and thought I needed a catheter. When the muscle relaxer failed to solve the problem, I asked my neurologist to prescribe a catheter.

The first time I used it, I thought I would die. Just the thought of putting something into an organ ordinarily associated with things coming out of it traumatized me. At least my wife was there to help. Her assurances that none of the men whom she had had to catheterize in the hospital had ever screamed in pain, let alone died, did nothing for my confidence.

"Yes, but I will," I countered, "I just know it."

With pursed lips, a sweaty brow, and a trembling hand, I set to the task. As my wife watched, I needed mountains of encouragement and reassurance, not to mention someone to revive me since I was certain I would pass out, I surveyed the problem. What first looked like a pencil-sized rubber tube grew before my very eyes to the girth of a fire hose.

"It'll never fit," I protested.

"Yes, it will," my wife assured me. "Just do it."

So, I inserted the catheter, millimeter by millimeter, no, micrometer by micrometer, all 20 yards of it. Then, suddenly, without any effort, I was urinating. What a strange feeling. I simply couldn't believe it. Utterly uncanny. And, it didn't even hurt.

In reporting my triumph to my neurologist, I said, "I always hoped to go to heaven, but I never thought I'd go penis first."

Unfortunately, I discovered that the first catheter I used was the wrong size. A stricture in my urethra necessitated the use of a smaller size catheter. The upshot of the episode is that I scratched my urethra. Consequently, the next time I urinated, the blood from the scratch turned my urine red.

"No more catheter for me!" I felt vindicated. "See, I told you it would kill me."

My self-righteousness lasted only until the day of my hemorrhoidectomy. To keep my veins open during the operation, the surgeon had an intravenous saline solution dripping into me. When I was wheeled into my room following the operation, my bladder was extremely full. Because of the trauma of the surgery, however, I was unable to urinate on my own. I asked for a catheter, and then announced that my wife would insert it.

"She can't do that," the nurse protested.

"Don't worry," I responded. "She's a doctor."

When she arrived, she drained 750 ml from me. More than 30,000 catherizations later and I haven't died yet. The episode of bladder problems taught me to be prepared to adapt to anything.

MS consumes physical and mental time. Physical time refers to the motor difficulties the illness creates. Everything takes longer. From dressing to eating to ambulating, I must plan for it to take longer than before. Planning notwithstanding, physical movement is still more stressful. Every movement takes a level of concentration that was almost unknown to me before. Nothing is spontaneous, everything requires calculation and intensity. It is commonplace for me to have half my dinner on the plate while everyone else has finished eating. Is it frustrating? Enormously. But, it is my reality. Responding with hostility only makes matters worse. My experience is that the harder I try, the harder things become. Or according to the old formula, "The harder I try, the gooder to be, the worser I am." Amen.

The stress is exhausting, further exacerbating the entire cycle. I marveled as my children bound up and down a flight of steps in magical movements. Knowing how difficult it became for me, I would tremble for their safety, forgetting, that my movements once were as casual as theirs. When I would attempt to climb stairs, I would try to remember my children, as well as how easy it used to be for me. It helped reduce the stress of the climb. At other times, however, I would hiss and spit, cuss and complain. I knew it wouldn't help, but it would act like a valve on a pressure cooker. In the current vernacular, it helps to "vent."

At the end of a day, I sometimes reflect on what I accomplished, and wonder, 'Is that all I did?' But, recounting the steps and the tedium it took to accomplish everything, I return to reality. Am I satisfied that I used twice as much energy to accomplish half as much as I once could? Of course not. It's tremendously annoying to be half as able as before. On the other hand, I am satisfied that it's still possible to do anything at all, regardless of how long it takes. Besides, it is not as if I have a choice. Accepting the illness is a constant enterprise for me. Patience makes swallowing the bitter pill of reality a bit easier.

Regrettably, MS consumes an inordinate amount of my attention. [In fairness, this was more true in the past when I was newly diagnosed, than in the present.] I refer to the hours spent reading, talking, and planning because of the illness. The number of hours weekly or monthly occupied with MS in one way or another seems countless. Whereas previously I could do things without a second thought, MS means that nothing is spontaneous or automatic any longer. Everything must be planned and plotted, usually well in advance and always in great detail. Life is no longer casual; it cannot be taken for granted at any stage. I recall the first time I told an old friend about the demands the illness was exacting. He was incredulous when he realized the extent to which he took his body for granted. So did I, at one time. So do we all. The challenge is to carry on, and to preserve our dignity.

The time MS absorbs also includes the extraordinary amount of rest it demands. Between the physical and mental stress, fatigue is a universal phenomenon. Rest becomes an essential part of life. Whether it is occasional naps or merely lying down, rest is an invaluable weapon in preserving my freedom. When to rest and for how long varies with a countless set of circumstances. As the kind of person who used to work constantly, the idea of stopping for anything, not to mention a nap in the middle of the day, was a major hurdle for me. Rest preserves my energy, as well as restores some I might have expended. There are days when I can go without a nap, and there are days when I need two. Whatever the demand, it is self-defeating to act as if I can do without it. So too, I require more sleep overnight. Eight hours is my goal, but I can occasionally get away with seven for a night or two. I have become extremely jealous of my resting and sleeping time. It pays dividends in the form of additional energy when I am diligent and attend to it. Contrarily, I hate myself and often vow never to take my body for granted again and deny it the rest it demands.

Having MS has also led me to contemplate my existence—past, present, and future. Memories of what used to be, and anxiety over what tomorrow will bring, consume inordinate amounts of time. Recalling what life was like before the illness, it is easy to slip into self-indulgence. But self-pity, hard as it is to resist, serves no purpose. If anything, it makes us despicable to others. Worrying about the future, although logical, perhaps even unavoidable, can change nothing. All it does is waste valuable time. This is not to suggest that I do not think of the future. Of course I do. But having learned how fragile life is, I do not count on it. For that matter, neither do I suffer fools lightly.

The time the illness has taken is the source of any anger I still harbor. While there are far more interesting, inviting, enlightening, and fulfilling things to do than think about the troubles of my body, MS necessitates my dwelling on them. The additional hours it takes to do the most mundane and ordinary tasks become a challenge and, when accomplished, a source of great triumph. How absurd to feel accomplished for doing something that other people do regularly and effortlessly. How horribly dull to be consumed by every imaginable triviality of physical existence all the time. Yet that is a cost of MS. If allowed, it will consume all my attention. To be sure, it cannot be denied. Beyond that, however, it deserves no more. In short, I won't allow it to define my life. Let me illustrate the wrong approach.

A neurologist I was seeing liked to refer to his patients as, 'Msers'. I refused the appellation on the grounds that I do not define my life according to my illness. I define myself as Popeye did quoted above, it just so happens that I have this crummy disease. I imagine what the epitaph on my gravestone would read if I defined myself by the illness. 'Here lies one good MSer', or 'He was a valiant cripple'. About the last thing I want people to remember me by is what MS has done to me.

Watching me struggle, people oftentimes ask, "How do you do it? Isn't it hard? Don't you get tired?"

Yes, it's hard. And yes, I get tired. but, I do it because there is no other way. It is as uncomplicated as that.

I'll be whipped before I'll permit an illness to control my life. This hyperbole exaggerates my hubris, for in many respects, the illness does control my life. Not being able to walk, I must rely on a wheelchair (they no longer have sedan chairs, dammit.). But, the focus I maintain is that walking, is not the defining characteristic of who I am. I will get where I am going one way or another. It will always take longer, and it will be more strenuous doing so, but I will get there. But, what if I just cannot do it? What if the body can be neither coaxed nor cajoled into doing what I want?

First, I delay in the hope that changing conditions will allow me to do what I intended. This occurs most often when I am overheated. Given enough time and cold liquid, I will eventually be physically able again. Second, if the disability seems more permanent, I can redefine my goal in a way that suits the new reality.

The clearest example of this is the challenge I faced attempting to drive. When I found myself lifting my right leg from the accelerator to the brake pedal, I decided that it was time to relinquish the wheel. Always having done the weekly grocery shopping, I was presented with a dilemma. My solution was to assume the responsibility for composing the weekly grocery list, and my wife shops for us. I was able to redefine my goal in a way that suits the new reality while still remaining a contributing member of the household.

Life does not always work out that neatly. Instances abound of goals that have been abandoned. As a student I painted and hung wallpaper during summers and on weekends for a living. My last 'tour of duty' was during the summer, 1978. Having to pay painters to do the work which people used to pay me to do, was a bitter pill to swallow. Further, having to suffer the work that some so-called artisan (too many of them aren't qualified enough to be called craftspeople) did, added salt to a wound. In the end, I am relieved to have the resources to be able to hire them. Similarly, I previously enjoyed refinishing antique furniture.

It was with a sense of accomplishment and joy that I would purchase someone's castoff at a garage sale, and make it beautiful again. My last job was a dresser I stripped and refinished in 1985 for our younger daughter. The accompanying night table still awaits refinishing. I used to delight in growing vegetables each summer. No longer. If I am on the ground these days, it is as a result of some accident, rather than by design. P

Do I miss painting, refinishing furniture, and gardening? You'd better believe I do. But I simply can't do them any more. So what? There still exist zillions of things I can do, that give me pleasure and satisfaction. Having tried only a small fraction of a tiny percentage of them, there remain plenty of options open to me yet. My challenge is finding the time and figuring out how to do them.

6

Going Public

Announcing to family and friends that I was diagnosed with multiple sclerosis was among the most difficult aspects of my illness. After all, nobody wants to be identified with a horrific illness. I certainly didn't. In retrospect it shouldn't have been, but that is the wisdom of hindsight.

My entire adult life people always knew me as a healthy, vigorous individual. More than being fiercely independent, I was proud of my independence. It was for that that I wanted to be remembered. MS changed all that. Now, I was saddled with an illness best known for destroying people's independence. Although my physical condition was only minimally altered—a slight limp on one side—I was confronted with the prospect of telling everyone that I was diagnosed with this horrendous crippling illness. I did not relish the responsibility of making my condition known.

Reputation, that is, what other people think of us, was difficult for me to ignore. Consequently, I must have acted as if I was responsible for contracting MS. My behavior was subconscious, because I never thought that contracting the illness was my fault. For whatever reason, though, I must have behaved as if it was something for which I could be held accountable. This foolish thinking controlled me.

'What will people think of me if I begin using crutches, never mind a wheelchair?' I wondered. 'Will they think I am giving in to MS? Oh no, I don't want to be thought of as weak, let alone be identified with those sick people.' I just need to be more determined.

This was an association I did not covet. It was better to keep it to myself, and 'admit' nothing. I didn't want people to think any less of me. So, for the longest time, I resisted doing anything that would reveal that I was suffering with MS. Worse, I resisted doing anything that would make my life easier. This is not to recommend reaching for all aids for disability immediately. They should be avoided, as long as possible. When the need arises, however, we should not hesitate to use them. That is easy for me to say today, but it was not always so.

Not long after I was diagnosed, a colleague's mother was diagnosed with terminal cancer. He and I spoke about my illness, and how to cope with a 'life sentence'. I recall telling him that I simply had to live with it. My focus was on making every day count as much as possible. Only after his mother died did he tell me that relating our conversations had been a great comfort in her final days. Many of her relatives blamed her for the cancer. For her part, she was feeling guilty for no reason.

When I began using crutches regularly (and subsequently I graduated to a wheelchair), my fears proved groundless. No one's opinion of me changed. Amazing. Why I thought they would less of me is indefensible. After all, when others begin using walking aids, my opinion of them doesn't change. Why should theirs of me?

Without admitting it, I was ashamed of having MS. That this was ridiculous goes without saying. What did I do to contract MS? Nothing. It was comparable to being ashamed of needing eyeglasses. In a society noted for the premium it puts on conformity and vigor, being different was a heavy burden. Nevertheless, sooner or later it would be discovered. The longer I waited, the more advanced the illness would become, and the more bizarre the rumors would be. So, as a matter of courtesy to those closest to me, as well as to squelch any whispers, I decided to 'go public'.

Publicly announcing my illness reminded me of what distinguishes couples who live together from those who get married. Many students have asked me the distinction between them, since they seem so much alike. My answer is that, yes, they look quite similar. When couples marry, however, they stand before their family and friends and publicly declare their commitment to one another for life. In other words, they put their good names behind the declaration of marriage. Couples who live together make no comparable public declaration. They stake nothing on their 'arrangement'. When their relationship ends, the individuals go their separate ways. When marriages fail, though, legal ramifications follow, and the mantle of divorce follows each party forever. My analogy, however, is flawed. Unlike marriage, I did not choose MS. It chose me.

Upon reflection, my resistance to using crutches or a wheelchair stemmed from sources deeper than mere concern for my reputation. As much as I told myself that I accepted the reality of MS, my actions belied that. I resisted letting the world see that I was afflicted with something that made me different, and, in a way less than other people. I emphasize 'in a way', because my differences from other people are limited to physical disabilities that restrict me from doing many things. They are of secondary importance, however, and far from the most important aspects of my life.

Would that I had focused on the important things from the start. Instead, I was concerned that people would judge me on the basis of ephemera. So, although I am acutely sensitive to the heat, I continued to wear a coat and tie to class. I count myself among the peculiar souls who actually enjoy neckties. Beyond that, I thought that looking professional was essential. Today, I wear a plain shirt—short sleeve, winter included. To my amazement, it has made no difference to my students. They still respect me. What I learned from this simple instance is that I cannot ignore my own particular needs, public conventions to the contrary. If it happens that others are offended, that is something they will have to endure. I cannot function in any other fashion.

Isn't it the essence of acceptance to admit that we people afflicted with MS are not like everyone else? That we are not able to do many things 'healthy' people can? But, who wants to admit that? We all want to be like our family, neighbors, and friends. It's our democratic right isn't it? Thomas Jefferson announced it in the Declaration of Independence.

We hold these truths to be self evident that all men are created equal, that they are endowed by their Creator with certain unalienable rights, that among these rights are life, liberty, and the pursuit of happiness.

Well, I was created equal, too, wasn't I? I have equal rights just like everyone else. But, the illness rendered me unable to exercise them. It makes me different. MS makes every sufferer different. Like it or not, in certain respects it makes us less than other people.

But who wants that? Alexis de Tocqueville, the French nobleman who visited the United States in the early 19th century, eloquently described the soul of democracy, its very essence. Equality, he says, is democracy's single most powerful impulse. We regard one another as equals. Even the slightest distinction makes us bristle. The most common distinction we refuse to tolerate is inequality in whatever form. Consider the 'rights' movements of our day: minority rights, women's rights, children's rights, gay rights, homeless rights, animal rights, and, yes, handicapped rights. Each and every 'rights' movement is a quest for equality, a plea that everyone acknowledge the equal status of a particular group. We want to treat everyone as if they are equal. Regardless of the cost, everyone wants, nay, demands equality.

Try as I might, I am not equal in certain fundamental respects. Physically, there are a million and one things I cannot do, and no amount of retrofitting can change that. To be sure accommodations can be made. Lower buttons on elevators, cut curbs, and handicapped parking spaces are adjustments that make life easier for me. I appreciate them, but it is a question of public policy to decide how much will be spent trying to make unequal individuals equal in an unequal world.

The Americans with Disabilities Act [ADA] is a national commitment to accommodations for the handicapped. It began as an attempt to incorporate the physically handicapped. Today, however, because no comprehensive definition of disability was ever established, everything imaginable is being claimed under the ADA. Claims are made for everything from obesity to psychological/psychiatric disorders (of which there are 374 listed in the latest DSM4). Back trouble is the only claim made more frequently. Only time will tell how far the nation will go in this regard. Meanwhile, I neither demand nor even expect special treatment. I appreciate it when it is there, but I also accept my being different.

Publicly acknowledging my inequality was a major hurdle. Tenaciously refusing to relinquish my independence, I did everything possible to avoid the mantle of cripple. Better to struggle with dignity than concede my need for assistance. What? Crutches? Me? Never! Don't want 'em. Don't need 'em. Not surprisingly, the idea of the crutches was not mine. It was the gentle, loving suggestions of my wife. She clearly saw the problem I refused to acknowledge.

Getting the crutches and using them, however, were two different things. When I started relying on crutches, I carried them in one hand in the morning, and used them as intended only late in the afternoon. My furtiveness was the manifestation of my self-consciousness over the need for assistance. When I carried the crutches people would ask whether I had hurt my leg. No, I would explain, it's just the MS giving me fits. To my surprise, no one reacted negatively. None thought any less of me. Life continued as before, except I sometimes used crutches. Today, it is a wheelchair, but I have detected no changes in people's opinions of me.

Using a wheelchair always struck me as the worst imaginable curse. Oh, no, to be confined to a wheelchair. How horrible! The chair, I discovered, is only a confinement if we can do more without it. But, when it allowed me to do more, my perception of it changed. Rather than a confinement, it became a liberation. I have looked at it that way ever since. Truthfully, I have a love/hate relationship with my wheelchair. On the one hand, it allows me to do considerably more than I could without it. On the other hand, sitting in it for too long makes me stiff and weak.

When I got the chair, my wife warned me that people would not see me in it. For whatever reason they would look past me as if I do not exist. She told me how people would ask an adult pushing a youngster in a wheelchair whether the child might want something to eat or drink. Never did it occur to them to ask the child whether he or she was hungry or thirsty. The scene has occurred to me many times. I will be attending a conference, and people I have known for years will walk past me as if I was not there. Perhaps, it's because I am sitting, and their focus is at a higher level. Or, possibly, it is a result of being unwilling to acknowledge the reality of a person in a wheelchair for fear that they might be there some day themselves. Whatever the explanation, I have learned to make my presence abundantly clear when I want to be acknowledged.

Being a cripple is a state of mind. To be sure, by most definitions I am a cripple. I do not contest that. But, I refuse to allow my physical limitations to control my life. They will slow me down, and interrupt things. Already, they have made life more complicated and difficult. I have had to change some plans, and abandon others. Yet, I see the challenge as one of staying ahead of the illness. In the same way a prize-fighter must always 'bob and weave' to avoid getting struck, so must I constantly move to stay out of harm's way. When the illness lands one, however, the only thing to do is to 'go with the punch', rest and regain enough strength to start bobbing and weaving again. Where the analogy breaks down, though, is in the ability of the fighter to strike back. My only weapons are defensive. I can only try to stay ahead of the illness by adapting and devising strategies to maximize my options. Fighting back is not an option.

I can say that one of my grudges with the illness is that although I suffer this dreadful condition, I don't have anything to show for it. To look at me, one sees the picture of health: no gnarled limbs, no drooping flesh, no palsy, no braces from hip to ankle. People say how well I look, while all I think is I wish it worked half as well as it looks.

MS has no explanation. We don't know why, or how we get it. Going public, nonetheless, is a giant step. Getting over the guilt of being sick is a crucial first step towards confronting any chronic illness. The less guilty we feel, the less guilty we act, and the less blame people will assign to us.

7

Drugs: Terrifying Terrific

People are terrified of drugs. Well, they should be. We all know stories of young people whose lives were destroyed by them. Week-in and week-out newspapers and the electronic media teem with accounts of crimes based on drug dependence. And, many of us know adults who have become addicted to prescription drugs. Although their lives may not have been destroyed, their dependence complicated things considerably.

In graduate school I recall how one of my professors would put his hand across his face every few minutes during class, and empty an eye-dropper full of antihistamines into his nose. Words cannot describe the snort to which all were subjected. Sadly, the man was captured in the cycle of antihistamine rebound.

In reaction to horror stories such as these, many people refuse all drugs. Several individuals I know go so far as to shun even Tylenol. This is perfectly ridiculous. For fear that they will become 'hooked' they needlessly suffer through all manner of discomfort. Clearly, this is not a case of ignorance being bliss. Quite the opposite. For fear of being unable to control themselves they do not take advantage of the benefits and relief medication has to offer.

I recall an example of a first-rate student I taught a couple years ago. 'Mary' worked especially hard. By every measure she was compulsive. She worked too many hours, slept hardly at all, and ate scarcely anything. Her mother was concerned that Mary was anorexic. Unable to complete all the work expected of her, Mary lost control one day, and had a nervous breakdown. A few days in the psychiatric ward showed her what people who truly need to be there look like. That scared her somewhat back to reality. Mary clearly needed counseling and probably medication. But she was petrified of taking drugs. In part, her reluctance was the stigma attached to taking psychiatric drugs. I spent nearly a dozen hours trying to persuade her to see a psychiatrist and, if need be, take medication. Happily, Mary's time in the hospital, and our lengthy conversations put her back in control. More to the point, she accepted the possibility of taking medication.

This is not a wholesale endorsement of either prescription, or over-the-counter [OTC] drugs. Most OTC drugs provide symptomatic relief, at best. They cure nothing, don't really change the course of an illness, and simply make us feel better. Sometimes they don't even do that. There's nothing wrong with feeling better; we all want that. Anti-inflammatory drugs and pain-killers can provide valuable relief. Nevertheless, they and other OTC drugs have their dangers. As with nose drops, or sprays, laxatives, or sleeping pills, they can be habit forming. Short of that, a psychological dependence can develop.

Many people are as afraid of prescription as of OTC drugs. A friend of mine became dependent on prescription tranquilizers. Detoxifying her took institutionalization for two months. The memories of the dependence left her scarred forever.

As one physician put it, "It's all poison, but with prescription medication, we take small enough amounts to be therapeutic."

Every medication, even the most benign, has side effects.

As a young man, I had no need of medication on a regular basis. When prescribed today, I do my best to stop taking it at the earliest recommended opportunity. Today, my MS require that daily I take seven prescriptions (14 pills). Additionally, I take two OTC medications (3 pills), and a couple of basic vitamins (5 pills). Until recently, I took twenty tablets of an additional medication daily. Today, the medication is now delivered directly into my central nervous system through a pump implanted under my skin. Not taking it by mouth, I avoid the systemic side effects. Consequently, I can take approximately

25 times as much as the maximum recommended dose with none of the usual side effects. Nothing about taking medication thrills me. I hate it. But being helpful to my condition, I take it. That's exactly the point: it helps, so I endure it.

The larger point is that medications should still be feared, but respected and even welcomed when necessary. Drugs can be our friends when prescribed and monitored by a physician. For several years I took an anti-spasticity pill every two hours, close to the maximum recommended dosage. During class I would pause, and pop a pill. To make light of it, I would look up at the class and declare, "I'm drug dependent, and I love it." Everyone would laugh, but the important point is that the medication was valuable. To function I needed it. I still do. At a rehabilitation facility I met a fellow sufferer who had been prescribed 4 times the recommended maximum dosage of anti-spasticity medication I had been taking. The side effects were so debilitating, that he opted to suffer the spasticity. It's boring and tedious to be always reaching for a pill, but the alternative is worse.

When I hear people complain about the high cost of drugs, I bristle. Is it worth a dollar or two to relieve a migraine? To prevent a seizure? To shrink the inflammation that causes the pain of arthritis? Just ask someone who suffers migraines, seizures, or arthritis. They'll all say it's worth that much, if not twice the price.

On average, it costs more than $250 million to develop, test, and market a new drug. While pharmaceutical companies receive a patent of 17 years over their products, effectively a monopoly, the reality is closer to 8-10 years. Mandated trials before a drug can be sold to the public are counted against a company's exclusive rights over it. During that time, the drug company must recover its costs, and collect enough revenue to begin research on new medication. Further, not every drug under development comes to fruition. Just because a company invests $80 million in no way ensures that a drug will be developed successfully, or turn a profit. It may never even be sold to the public at all. If capitalism means anything, it signifies that all investments must be considered a risk. As such, if a drug is successfully developed, the pharmaceutical house is entitled to reap the profits.

Conversely, regardless of the amount of money or research invested, a failed attempt at developing a new drug returns nothing. We've all heard the grumbling over the 'obscene' profits of the drug companies. Consider, however, when was the last time we heard a syllable of sympathy for the millions of dollars and years of research that went for naught? I do not weep for the poor, downtrodden, drug companies, but neither do I begrudge them their profits. Most of them, in fact, will provide free medication for the indigent.

For a wide variety of reasons, many people have turned to alternative medicine. Whether in reaction to the high cost of drugs, or an ideological commitment to 'organic' living, people seek herbs, fungi, vitamins, magic pyramids, or almost any other conceivable source of magic remedy for their ills. There is an unspoken hubris behind this.

"I'm going to solve this problem using natural remedies. All the conventional research overlooked the real solution hanging out right there in nature."

Sad to say, this arrogance is generally expensive, foolish, and dangerous.

First, none of these secret remedies has been subjected to rigorous scientific tests. If they have positive effects, we don't know why, or exactly how to get the same results. To the extent something is efficacious, we have no way of knowing whether it was the natural remedy or the placebo effect. It amazed me to learn that upwards of 30% of all drug trials look successful only because of the placebo effect. Thinking a 'medication' will make us better, our condition improves.

In a recent trial my neurologist gave me an injection that had remarkably positive results. Suspecting that it was attributable to the placebo effect, he gave me a mock injection the next day. When it had no effect on my condition, we had a reasonable basis for concluding that the real injection had worked. Fearing that I might be angry for the deception, my neurologist apologized. I thanked him for the trial because it proved that the effect of the injection was genuine.

Rarely are comparable trials done on natural remedies. Anecdotal accounts are cited as proof of their effectiveness. Natural remedies are generally justified by individual subjective testimonials. Advertisements tout case after case of individuals who 'run faster and jump higher' because of a secret potion (or was it a secret lotion?). Yet, it is astounding to see how much better people do if they think that a particular pill will improve their abilities. Peer review of natural remedies doesn't exist, and all 'research' on them must be considered anecdotal. We have no way of knowing whether or not a natural remedy is actually working to relieve our condition.

Second, natural remedies lack consistency. A friend brought me a Kombucha mushroom from which I was supposed to brew a tea with extraordinary powers. The tea is brewed by soaking the mushroom in ordinary black tea enriched with sugar. Its healing powers promise relief for cancer, arthritis, multiple sclerosis, and anything else that might ail a body. The maturity of the mushroom, the concentration of the tea, the duration the mushroom is to soak, and the amount of tea to be consumed are all unregulated. Two weeks after bringing me the mushroom, my friend discovered that she was allowing the mushroom to soak in the sugar solution too long. Consequently, the tea she was drinking was fermented. I don't know what it did for her arthritis, but after a glass of 'hard' tea, nothing bothered her. Conceivably, the tea might well have helped her, but, then again, it might as easily have been an incantation by the tooth fairy.

Third, 'natural' remedies are unspecific. It's rather like shooting squirrels with a shotgun. We might succeed in killing the squirrel, but we might also kill ten birds, seven chipmunks, a raccoon, and Uncle Henry along the way. A panorama of different illnesses is treated with the same antidote. Drugs, by contrast, are developed to treat very specific problems. This is not to say that the same drug cannot have unexpected benefits. They do. For example, an anti-high blood pressure medication turned out to be a valuable anti-migraine treatment.

Fourth, drug interactions are never discussed. Ginkgo biloba can interact with blood thinners to heighten their effect. The result can be disastrous. The bottle we are sold never contains a warning to that effect. This is typical of natural remedies.

Fifth, 'natural' remedies are presumed to be safe until proven otherwise. The amino acid L-tryptophan has the effect of making one very drowsy. Sold as a sleeping pill, it was discovered that the medium on which it was being grown contained a potentially fatal bacterium. Until people died, it was thought safe. Comparable trust in drugs does not exist. Rather, they are tested almost to a fault, before they are approved for to the public.

The pro-nature approach also inaccurately posits a basic tension between nature and medicine. Fundamentally, modern medicine refines nature to make it regular and consistent. For example, digitalis, a medication to regularize heartbeats, is derived from the foxglove plant. The problems of how much of the plant should be consumed, how mature it should be, which parts are to be consumed, how often they should be taken, and so forth are solved by refining foxglove plants into consistent tablets. Medicine essentially improves on nature.

A number of years ago, Sandoz (a Swiss pharmaceutical house) discovered cyclosporine, a powerful anti-rejection drug in a handful of dirt. Like all the major drug companies, they have a standing policy of requiring their representatives to bring back some dirt from wherever they go. Today, cyclosporine is used following transplant operations to suppress the body's inclination to reject the new organ. Had Sandoz not developed it, cyclosporine would still be hidden in the dirt. Could someone eat a handful of the 'right' dirt following a transplant, and not reject a new organ? Perhaps, but I would more likely attribute the results to chance.

I recall how my neighbor was too cheap to visit a doctor or buy any medication. Whenever he fell ill with a cold or virus, Ray would allow a piece of cheese to grow mold, and then eat it. He thought he had a cheap source of penicillin. Who knows what he was eating? But after washing it down with a case of beer, he didn't especially care. Happily, I moved 300 miles away before I could witness any long-term consequences of his lunacy.

Finally, there is an underlying assumption that all things 'natural' are to be preferred to things that mankind has done. This ideology overlooks the entire spectrum of instances where nature has proven hostile to mankind, and where human artifice has been beneficial. Just to take two obvious examples: smallpox and polio. Both have been rendered virtually extinct thanks to vaccines. Without the efforts of medical research, we would still be suffering the ravages of these two. Regrettably, not all of medicine's efforts are so successful. As it is, most chronic illnesses still remain a mystery. Yet, even short of conquering MS, medicine has rendered my life with them eminently more bearable.

8

Depression

Depression is a natural accompaniment to MS. It could hardly be otherwise. As the illness eats away at the body, it exacts an even greater toll on the spirit. There is simply no escaping the illness. Every minute of every day I am reminded that I have MS. Each action requires an effort of the soul comparable to the physical effort required of the body. Lurking in the background is the gnawing question: will I be able to do everything I ask of my body today? Or, how much longer will I be able to carry on as I do now? Every change in my condition demands a new effort to respond. When emotional resources are exhausted, when I feel beaten to a frazzle, my body chemicals become unbalanced. I become depressed.

Depression manifests itself in a myriad of ways. There can be changes in all of life's basic patterns. Appetite will frequently diminish. Alternatively, some individuals will eat compulsively. Emotions are sometimes uncontrollable, everything from snapping at everyone around, to weeping at the drop of a hat. Emotions are right on the surface. Ambition diminishes, as does self-confidence. Making a decision becomes difficult, if not impossible. Meeting life's responsibilities, whether at home or work is done poorly, if at all. Falling asleep (or back to sleep after awakening during the night) takes longer and longer, if it ever occurs at all. Conversely, some depressed individuals use sleep as an escape. I know of one woman who would pack her children off to school in the morning, then go back to bed. Good news brings almost no relief, while a heightened sense of guilt and shame hangs over life. There is a constant feeling of helplessness and hopelessness.

For fourteen years I watched my level of disability increase. It was not a steady progression, but a series of plateaus, each at a higher level of disability than the last. For the first several years, life continued largely unchanged. Nearly three years after being diagnosed, I walked more than a mile with my year old daughter in a back carrier. Other activities were fundamentally unaffected: swimming, cooking, gardening, eating, handwriting, driving, dressing. As the fifth year approached I waited anxiously. This a benchmark year. The research indicates that if an MS sufferer is walking after five years, they are likely not to have to rely on a wheelchair. As I was walking after five years, albeit with Canadian crutches, I cheered inside. While I thought I was home free, it did not last. Reluctantly, I yielded to the necessity of a wheelchair. Around the same time, I realized my legs were not strong enough to drive responsibly. Lifting my right foot from the accelerator with my right hand, and placing it on the brake pedal was not safe. I relinquished the wheel to my wife.

No longer able to walk much, I was still able to stand for long periods of time. I continued to do most of the cooking at home. Not only is cooking among my favorite avocations, but I felt that I was making a significant contribution to the household. Dressing became more challenging, but a loving wife helped me. My teaching duties continued, but now pushing the wheelchair became more difficult. Getting to a standing position was a greater challenge, but many helpful students were always willing to lend a hand. My community volunteer activities continued, although I now attended meetings in my wheelchair. Swimming was still possible for me (I revel in the memory of swimming laps beside my older daughter), but climbing up and down the pool ladder became more dicey. Nevertheless, I was sufficiently self-assured of my abilities that I accepted the presidency of my synagogue.

Summers have been particularly difficult for me, with MS making me weak from the heat and humidity. Never was this truer than during the summer of 1994. During July, the twenty-five year old air conditioner in our house gave up the ghost. Although a local company installed a new unit, it was not before the temperature in the house reached a steamy 86 degrees. Weak does not begin to describe how debilitated I was. A month later I slipped while pouring a kettle of boiling water and my hand hit a red-hot burner. With third degree burns on my left hand, my cooking career was over. Upon removing the dressing the first time, I came within a hairbreadth of passing out at the sight. The burns shook my confidence as much as they disabled my hand. My cooking days were over. Meanwhile, academic year 1994-95 was the first time I taught from the wheelchair. While the students were unaffected by my being seated, it wore on me.

"What has become of me," I wondered, "that I can't even stand in front of a class?"

Would that I had paid more attention to the students, and less to myself. By the middle of 1995, I realized that I was grossly overextended. Approaching the end of my third year as president of the synagogue, my duties included responsibility for the budget. As the end of the fiscal year approached, a deficit loomed. While there were other officials in the synagogue, none felt a responsibility for the budget like I did. Additionally, whenever anything went wrong, I was always called. Beyond presiding over the synagogue, I was nearing the conclusion of my seventh and eighth years respectively on the boards of directors of the Syracuse Hebrew Day School and the Syracuse Jewish Community Center, respectively. Mentally and emotionally drained, I skipped meetings. My absences only contributed to feelings of inadequacy.

Beyond the burden of these three communal duties, my house had become a greater strain on me. For eight years I had negotiated a flight of stairs to enter my house, as well as to get to my desk. As the years passed, they became a progressively greater challenge. To solve the problem, we had a stair lift installed. After using it successfully for two years, a decline in my condition made getting on and off the lift a chore, and a peril. I would stand at the top of the stairs and wonder, 'Is this the time when I go crashing to the bottom?'

I was exhausted in every imaginable way. Waking up in the middle of the night became commonplace. To make matters worse, I was having difficulty falling back to sleep. The problems of the day would consume me. Try as I might, I could neither solve them, nor clear them from my thoughts. Hours would pass, exhaustion would overcome me, and I would fall back to sleep. In the morning I would spend the day tired. The more fatigued I became, the less I was able to do. Worse, my ambition and confidence were spent as well.

When the cycle continued, my wife encouraged me to tell my neurologist. He prescribed an antidepressant, Prozac. Of course I had heard of it, but disdained those who took it. Despite feeling perfectly awful, I was still not ready to admit that I was depressed. I labored under the foolish misconception that depression is a function of a weak character. The only remedy someone who was depressed needs, I thought, is to clench his jaw, grasp the nettle firmly, and buck up. How naïve, judgmental, and wrong I was.

The medication I took for depression had a half-life in excess of two weeks. Accordingly, it had almost no effect on me for almost a month. Meanwhile, I found that my bladder would only hold 3 to 4 ounces of urine before demanding to be emptied. This annoyed and distressed me because I was accustomed to catheterizing 6 to 10 ounces. And, my otherwise equable wife was growing short with me. Then, she came home from the office one day with news for me.

"I was reading the PDR [Physician's Desk Reference] today," she announced, "and discovered that 4% of all patients who take Prozac develop urinary urgency."

No sooner did I learn that then I asked my neurologist for a different antidepressant. Before changing, however, I first had to evacuate my body of a remaining Prozac. This was necessary because each drug has its own side effects. It is essential not to overlap them. I stopped taking Prozac before I thought it had had a chance to be fully effective.

Life was still perfectly awful for me. I had no ambition, nor was I satisfied with anything I attempted.

Then, I received a phone call from a psychologist/friend of mine. To my utter amazement, he talked to me as another professional. For 30 minutes he treated me better than I had been treating myself. The conversation left me walking on air. I determined that I did not want to be depressed. So there! Take that, hrumpf! Little did I know that my bravado was the result of the Prozac actually being efficacious. It just happened to coincide with the psychologist's call. The antidepressant made it possible for me to cope with life's wrinkles. No longer did every molehill take on the proportions of a mountain. My motivation returned. The weight of the world was lifted from my shoulders. I stopped chewing my family's heads off at every turn. Hard as it was to believe, I no longer thought I was an altogether worthless human being.

Interestingly, the Prozac didn't make everything better. Contrary to popular characterizations, anti-depressants are not 'happy pills'. They aren't intended to have that effect. They will not chase away the blues. Rather, they make it possible for us to make our lives better.

A few days later, the Prozac fell below the therapeutic level. My determination crumbled, my confidence dissolved, and a black cloud descended over me. My depression returned with a vengeance. Luckily, I was already familiar with it, so I was able to recognize it. I still felt horrendous, but I knew that an antidepressant would relieve my condition. Until I could get back to a therapeutic level of antidepressant in my blood I was able to cope with the depression. The larger lesson I derived was that depression is genuine. It cannot be defeated by determination or will. Rather, it is a function of a chemical imbalance in the brain that can be treated successfully with medication. Until it happened to me, I didn't believe it was real.

While I never contemplated suicide I can understand why so depressed people do. Never did I feel so helpless and useless as during the depths of depression. I had always fashioned myself to be a strong individual, capable of meeting all of life's challenges. When life got to be too much for me, I was relieved that others less arrogant than me had figured out ways to treat it.

Arguably, among the greatest tragedies of our day is the individual whose depression goes untreated. Repeatedly, accounts fill the media of terminally ill individuals who opt for suicide. Upon autopsy, they are found only to be suffering from depression. To me, that is the very definition of tragedy.

9

Don't Believe It! People Still Care

We take it for granted these days that people only care for themselves. Stories of the woman who is accosted before dozens of onlookers, or the purse snatching that occurs on a busy street are painful reminders that we no longer care for one another. That we take these things for granted has been cited as an example of the extent to which our society has become coarsened and corrupted. Senator Daniel Patrick Moynihan described this acceptance in an article entitled, 'Defining Deviancy Down'. He painfully articulates how we look passively, almost nonchalantly, upon what used to horrify us. In response, Charles Krauthammer wrote, 'Defining Deviancy Up', in which he shows how the media have found the same deviant actions, previously attributed to the lowest stratum of society, prevalent among the highest. AIDS, murder, and all manner of corruption are present among the most prominent stars are singled out as examples of how no one is immune from these perversities. So, from either direction a general lack of mutual concern seems to be the watchword of the day. Presidential inaugural addresses by Presidents Bush and Clinton to the contrary notwithstanding, the pleas for mutual caring seem to have fallen on deaf ears.

Senior citizens speak wistfully of the 'good old days' when people did care, but that is a bygone era. The number of times, elderly friends have lamented how everything these days is not as good as years ago seems innumerable. It is arguable whether this is attributable to romantic nostalgia or an unwillingness to accept the progress time has made. Regardless, too many of us liken remembrances of our youth with either quality or superiority. Too often we are unprepared to realize that the goodness of the good old days, is not quite as we remember them.

By contrast, I firmly believe that our lives today can be as happy as we choose to make them. Sure, we are saddled with this crippling disease, but that does not make us useless. Neither does it render us less than human. Sure, we hear of the occasional outpouring of concern for the child who falls into an open well. There are also the heroic efforts of a passerby who risks his life by diving into the icy waters of the Potomac River to save the victims of a plane crash. Events like these stand out, though, because they are the exception and not the rule.

Don't believe the doomsayers. People really do care. I would not have guessed this to be so, had the circumstances of my life not demonstrated it time and again. From the time I began using Canadian (forearm) crutches, life has been a repeated succession of unsolicited acts of kindness. More often than I care to remember, I would fall down. A pebble would lurk like a boulder threatening to upend me. A crack in the sidewalk would wait like a snare ready to grab my ankles and hurl me to the cement. A carpet, innocent as it might appear, would sit like a trip wire eager to send me reeling. Too often, I would find myself looking up from the ground rather than down at it. The combination of being startled and jolted would leave me unable to move. Before I could even catch my breath, there would be some stranger standing over me with hand outstretched.

"Are you all right?" he would worriedly ask.

"Yes, dammit." I was livid for having been so clumsy as to lose another round with gravity.

"Let me give you a hand." And, before I knew it, one or two people would be lifting me up.

Once a utility company employee screeched his truck to a halt when he saw me prone on the side of the road. He pulled me out of the grass, dusted me off, and then, contrary to company policy, offered me a ride. I recall being so taken aback by both having fallen and his kindness that I declined his offer.

Another time, a young couple saw me crash to the subway platform in the Washington, DC Metro. In a rush to get off the train before the doors ate my leg, I lost my footing. My foolish delight at thinking I had outsmarted the train was quickly overcome by my humiliation from the ignominious defeat that left me face down on the platform. A young couple quickly came to my rescue. Each took an arm, righted me, and retrieved my crutches. Only when they were satisfied that I was all in one piece did they bid me farewell.

Among the countless such instances, one stands out from the rest. That was the day I emerged from the Washington Metro into a pouring summer rain. Faced with a ten-minute walk to reach my conference, I was in a quandary. For most people either an umbrella or a raincoat would have solved the problem, but holding a crutch in each hand and carrying an umbrella is a feat no one has figured out how to do. Wearing a raincoat was out, too, because of my sensitivity to the heat. Summer being the bane of MS sufferers, I chose to take my chances. As I paused under an awning contemplating how to dance between the raindrops, a woman appeared beside me, umbrella in hand. That this perfect stranger was willing to get half-wet so that I would only get half-wet, touched me. Not only that. As I was in desperate need of a restroom, she was kind enough to find one for me in a bookstore/coffee bar. After waiting patiently for me, she escorted me to the nearest bus stop, stood with me until it arrived, guided me up the steps, and then pressed the 'exact change' into my hand! For his part, the bus driver made an unsolicited, unauthorized, illegal stop directly in front of the hotel where the conference was being held. So that I would not get drenched, he violated company and city rules. It must have been a sight for all the people at the conference to see me walking on air. I simply could not believe the unsolicited kindness of these two strangers. I'll never forget either of them.

Being a cripple is not a joy. As with everything else in my life, however, I have attempted to learn from it. Here I paraphrase Will Rogers. He used to say that he'd never met a man he didn't like. Sad to say, I've met many a man I didn't like. But I've never met a man (or woman) from whom I haven't learned. Having limited use of my legs has given me the opportunity to discover that people do still care. It has made my life considerably more pleasant and easier. My most fervent hope is that I might be able to help others in some small way comparable to the help I've been shown.

10

From Independence to Dependence and Back Again

Before taking ill, I prided myself on being fiercely independent. Isn't that the American way? The rugged individualist spirit enshrined in the Declaration of Independence? The pioneer spirit that conquered the 'Wild West'? My independence began early, as a matter of necessity.

After my mother died when I was 12, my father hired housekeepers and baby-sitters for my two younger sisters (ages 9 and 4) and me. That lasted until he went bankrupt a year and a half later. The responsibility of housekeeper, baby-sitter then devolved to me (age 14). That I knew scarcely anything about cooking, cleaning, and washing didn't matter. In retrospect the idea of burdening a 14-year-old boy with those responsibilities horrifies me. That same year I bought a newspaper route, and began doing odd jobs for neighbors, friends, and relatives. I don't mean to exaggerate my role. My father still paid the rent, but I contributed for the family groceries. As well, I split my earnings with him to pay for gas for his car.

A year after my father remarried, I went to college, but received no financial support from home. At the end of my first year, I persuaded my father and his wife to declare me financially independent. That I was also suffering pangs of adolescence contributed to my discomfort. Shortly thereafter, I left home. During the remaining 3 years as an undergraduate, I worked two jobs to support myself. As a graduate student, I worked as a teaching assistant during the academic year, and a painter and paperhanger during the summers. At the end of graduate school, I typed my Ph.D. dissertation myself. The first summer I did not work was 1979.

After moving to Syracuse (September 1980), I became friends with a man who effectively gave me a three-family house. Two of the apartments required repairs, but he agreed to help me fix everything. Whatever needed doing, we did it: plastering, painting, carpentry and plumbing. I delighted in the sense of accomplishment it gave me. Painting and paperhanging are quite the same, as gardening. You can see the fruits of your labor. Teaching, by contrast, has few tangible results. Occasionally, students do well and go to law school, others request recommendations, and some thank me for the course they concluded. They, however, are the exception. For the most part, the rewards of teaching are never seen.

To be sure, I exaggerate how independent I was. Cars are a limit I readily acknowledge. God made 'em, let Him fix 'em, is my approach. Nonetheless, I prided myself on doing a wide variety of activities.

As the poet John Donne wrote, "No man is an island unto himself."

Until we reach a certain maturity, or until MS or some other chronic illness afflicts us, it is just a poem. That's when the day when we cannot do everything ourselves arrives. It began for me when I could no longer take long walks. Neither could I do the repairs my home required. My dependence continued to grow. Today I need a great deal of assistance, more than I care to contemplate. My wife helps me dress and undress. My daughters push me hither and yon, and bring me whatever I need. Friends do all manner of things, from fixing lunch to helping me in the bathroom. They, very kindly, drive me wherever I need to go. At school students push me from my office to class, and my secretary does everything from opening my mail to pushing me to the department office. Strangers are enormously helpful, too. Countless times they have opened doors, given me a push, transferred me from car to wheelchair or the reverse, or offered to bring me food or drink.

Going from independence to dependence can be very depressing. I still don't like it, but I have no choice. No amount of kicking, screaming, or gnashing my teeth will make me as independent as I was before. As my level of disability progressed, however, it occurred to me that I would still have to be responsible for my own happiness. I don't believe anyone owes me anything. This applies equally to family, friends, and total strangers. For them to help me, they have to want to do it. My responsibility is to be the kind of person whom people want to help. This is not meant to sound crass and calculating. It isn't. Rather, I simply try never to act as if I expect the help. When it is forthcoming, I am as grateful and appreciative as I can be. The more important point is that no one can make us happy. We have to do that for ourselves.

Maintaining my independence despite considerable physical dependence demands significant mental effort. I do my best not to define myself in physical terms and all that that entails. That I require a great deal of assistance goes without saying. But, that alone says nothing about so many other aspects of me. I can still be a warm, loving husband, and a tender father. None of these things requires much physical effort.

Likewise, I am still a challenging teacher. A few years ago, in fact, I was told that a female student I had never met was so terrified of me, that she was too scared even to walk past my office door. This is not a reputation I covet, but I do feel responsible for maintaining the quality of the students' education. They generally rise to the challenge, acquit themselves admirably, and enjoy my classes.

I remain a dedicated friend primarily through heartfelt conversations. Whether in person, via e-mail, by letters, or on the telephone, finding common grounds for discussions delights me. Being fully, physically able would help, but not being so does not deprive me of the most important, defining aspects of who I am.

Last, and perhaps most sustaining, I am a student. For more than 30 years I have actively studied politics: first as an undergraduate, then as a graduate student, and finally as a professor. Through books, journals, radio, the Internet, or television, I am always hungering after information and analyses of the world of politics. Just studying, though, has never been enough to sustain me. Being that one-dimensional strikes me as horribly dull.

My ultimate goal, rather, is to be the best person possible in every respect: husband, father, friend, and so forth. Succeeding at that enterprise is a life's work. Whether I have accomplished my goal may best be measured by the effort invested, rather than the results achieved. It begins by my being as attentive as possible to everything and everyone around me. Whenever I am shown consideration, caring, generosity, or compromise, I attempt to learn from it, and incorporate the admirable characteristics and behaviors I see in others. Conversely, I try to avoid the mistakes I see others make.

I do not pretend to have succeeded in my efforts. But, by trying to improve myself, I am constantly attempting to enrich and improve what I bring to the relationships in my life. That is the key. The quality of our relationships is arguably the prime determinant of our happiness. Nothing else is as fulfilling or as satisfying. By contrast, I have seen many people who move to a different city in the belief that their happiness depends fundamentally on their location. How misguided they are. Establishing and maintaining a family and friendships require several things.

First, we cannot think only of ourselves. Individuals with MS are especially susceptible to this. It is only natural that our chronic illness should be a constant preoccupation. But, does anyone else care about it as much as we do? No, of course not, because no one experiences the illness with the same degree of intimacy as us. It reminds me of the time when I was a landlord. No tenant ever cared for an apartment like I did, because I had a proprietary interest in it that they didn't. With nothing invested in the building, maintaining it was not a priority to them. MS is, first and foremost, my own problem. I cannot reasonably expect others to care as much about it as I do. Few things are more boring than someone whose conversations are always about themselves.

Those relationships are sure not to last. Others' welfare must also be our concern to establish a common bond for a lasting relationship.

Second, we need to find common interests with other people. Our mutual illness is a logical beginning, but if it goes no further, it will likely end there. There need to be more points of intersection to maintain a relationship. Whether it is hobbies, family, reading, religion, or a host of other things, we need issues we can share in common with others. They must be the foundation for establishing and maintaining a friendship.

Third, the ancient Greek philosopher Aristotle described true friends as those people who try to outdo one another in virtue. So it must be with us. We have to work at doing the best things for our family and friends. Our physical disabilities limit how much we can do, but that is not an excuse for doing nothing. A letter, a greeting card, an e-mail, or a phone call are within everyone's reach. A visit is better still, but may not be possible. Caring and concern don't cost anything. Relationships are a 'two way street' that demand contributions by both parties.

11

Strife of the Spirit

By chipping away at our bodies, MS reaches for our souls. The constant battle to maintain our physical existence inevitably involves a strife of the spirit. Many a time when I would struggle up a flight of stairs, I would repeat inwardly, 'It's all just mental; there's no reason I can't make it'. That I would not always succeed is testament to the limits of this 'mind over matter' philosophy. I will not recount what I would say when I conceded that it's not all in my head. [Actually, it is all in my head because that's what MS attacks, but that's beside the point.]

MS is a constant test. Our will to continue is challenged daily, if not hourly. Capitulating, however, is not an option for me. It never has been. I would not be able to respect myself if I gave my life over to the illness. Instead, I live as if I am prepared to die at any moment, confident that I will leave a good legacy behind.

My blithe attitude did not come easily. When first diagnosed I was unsure how long I had to live. The future was uncertain, and I did not want to count on anything. My neurologist joked about being afraid to buy green bananas, but the reality was that I was concerned about buying too many weeks worth of groceries at once. More than anything, the uncertainty terrified and wore on me. How could it be otherwise? I was fearful at every step. The only certainty in my life was a dreadful illness. How could I go on with this awful sentence? The inherent danger was that I would spend my life waiting for the other shoe to drop.

Somewhere along the line, I remember neither when nor why, it occurred to me that I could not spend my life raging against something, in my case MS. That would constitute surrender, because I would have allowed the illness to dictate the terms of my life. No illness deserves that. I'm more important than an illness. While all this sounds cavalier, it really is not. It is a reflection of my priorities. Dealing with my illness is not a matter of choice. It never is. Doing so, in fact, is little short of an annoyance, albeit a demanding one. It is not a calling to manage the illness; it's just a nuisance. I treat it as no more than that. How do I keep fighting as I witness the circle of my life growing smaller? Confronting MS, more than anything else, is a psychological enterprise. We must learn how to be our best selves despite the illness. That is a tall order. Ironically, the will to fight begins with what appears to be capitulation.

First, I had to accept the reality of MS and all that it implies. The simple, unpleasant reality is that I am sick today, I will be sick tomorrow, and so on for the rest of my life. Nothing good can be said about this situation, but it is a reality I can not deny. Sure, there are better and worse days, but the bottom line is there is always a cloud hanging over me. Being completely well is not one of m options. Accepting that reality is the first step in living up to life's potential. In a sense, this is really no different than the limits each of us is born with. I might have dreamed of playing professional basketball, but my being less than 5 ft. 6 in. tall ruled that out. Reconciling ourselves to the limits of our genetic composition is something we all do, but accepting the limits of MS is considerably more difficult. In that case we must reconcile ourselves to losing something we once had. And unlike dying gray hair another color, the losses MS inflicts are generally final.

I frequently put this problem to my students. They are willing to permit the Supreme Court to identify new rights. Whether it is the right of women to an abortion, or the right to privacy of couples, they are all for it. By contrast, they are unwilling to allow the Supreme Court to withdraw any of the rights they have identified. For us, the situation is comparable, but worse: we are forced against our will to relinquish something we had.

We are all accustomed to having a certain measure of control over our lives, but MS doesn't respect that. I find myself at the mercy of a horrendous illness. In varying degrees and in a myriad of ways, it regularly reminds me of my vulnerability, and my mortality. Although I was healthy all my life, I now had to adjust to the reality of being ill. And to think, I didn't do anything to get this way. What a bitter pill to swallow. But, swallow it we must. There simply is no reasonable alternative. Of course, I could 'throw in the towel', but that is the coward's way out.

I am reminded of the early days of my marriage. I would muse with my new wife about the things that I once owned, but which went with my first wife when we were divorced. Whenever we would happen across a household item in a store I would say, "I used to have one of those." We would both laugh, knowing exactly what it meant. The reality was that I did not have it any longer, and would never get it back. Fretting about it was useless, and foolish. As such, it would serve no earthly purpose. Mourning for the costs of MS are quite the same. It is like crying over spilled milk. The only choice is living within the limits the illness sets.

As to the future, I dream of it, but count on nothing. When I was diagnosed, I cried on my wife's shoulder that I always wanted to be a grandfather. Who knows if I will ever see that day? There are still courses I want to teach, and projects I want to accomplish. Whether I will ever have the wherewithal to do these things is impossible to know. None of us knows when or where the next tragedy will strike. Yet we still drive the streets despite the fear of drunk drivers, and we still buy lottery tickets, even if hitting the jackpot is a remote possibility. Planning allows me to get beyond the travails of today, beyond the illness. All this being so, why does MS intimidate us so? Perhaps it is a painful reminder that we are not in control of our lives. The challenge of living with MS is maintaining our identity. Only if we do that, can we confront the illness.

I reflect my disdain for the illness in my response to inquiries about how I am doing. Ordinarily, I respond in one of two ways.

At times I say, "I can't complain."

This always stymies people.

"What do you mean, you can't complain?" they respond. "You're in a wheelchair, and I remember when you could walk or run."

"Listen," I retort, "I could be fertilizer. What do I have to complain about?"

Or, if the MS is giving me fits, I'll say, "I'm fine, but my body stinks. We're not talking these days; it's angry at me for something, but it refuses to say what."

This reflects my refusal to allow the illness to define me. I see the two of us as independent, entities that happen to occupy the same body. My familiarity with the illness and my body make these episodes of distinguishing between body and self, less necessary than before. Nevertheless, I acknowledge that the illness has the upper hand. My responsibility, like a prizefighter, is to keep 'bobbing and weaving', always trying to keep from being struck a crushing blow.

There are times when I cannot avoid dealing with it, body and soul. There isn't a single minute in any day when I am not aware that I have MS. That is an unavoidable necessity. Even in the darkest moments, I do my damnedest not to make the illness the focus of my life. There is no future in it.

When hospitalized, for example, I try especially hard to assist by roommate in any way possible. Whether it is encouragement or small talk, I do whatever I can to make life more bearable. Recently, my roommate who was developmentally disabled, was terrified of needles. When his intravenous needle had to be changed, I beckoned him to count with me to 50. I began, "One," and he would repeat, "One." By the time we got to 30, the IV had been changed, and he didn't even know it. I felt gratified that I had the opportunity to help someone.

I have a lot to live for. We all do. Actually, I consider myself the luckiest guy in the world. I have a wife for whom I want to be a good husband. Since taking ill, I have added two wonderful daughters for whom I want to be a fine father. (And I thought that MS was a challenge!) I have students whom I want to teach, studies I want to do, books I want to read, civic and religious responsibilities I want to fulfill. There is a person I want to be. In the face of all these rich and rewarding possibilities, I reject the idea of allowing the disease to define my life.

Perhaps it is a function of my being the pre-law adviser at school. Students who apply to law school must prepare a personal statement, an explanation of what distinguishes them from the other thousands of applicants. They are hard pressed to think of anything until I would challenge them with a question or two.

"What made you who you are? Was it a triumph or a tragedy? Your father, mother, a grandparent, another relative, or a friend? A book or television show?"

The same proposition applies to MS sufferers. Each of us is distinguished in ways we don't appreciate. We need to realize that we each have contributions to make to this world. Being a cripple is not among them.

I don't refer to myself as 'handicapped' or 'disabled', even though according to all conventional definitions, I am both. I tell my students they are free to call me a cripple or a gimp if they choose, but not to refer to me as handicapped. Being handicapped is a state of mind, whereas being crippled is a condition of body. I am not handicapped. I am driven to accomplish many things, and become the person I am not yet. Am I a cripple? Sure, but so what?

Dealing with the needs of my body in no way makes me a better person. It does not enrich my life to have mastered the challenge of everyday living. At most, I am functional. Life has far more interesting and fulfilling enterprises than the problems of day to day existence. Keeping my focus on what I want to be, and what I dream about accomplishing, puts the illness in perspective. MS is just another stumbling block in the path of my life.

William Faulkner put it well.

'Your outside is just what you live in, sleep in, and has little connection with who you are.'

12

Confronting MS

MS, I discovered, plays by its own rules. Accordingly, it must be confronted in its own way. We cannot fight it as an ordinary illness. For those of us who have always been accustomed to being in control, this is a difficult lesson to learn. If anything, we must be accept MS as our master. No amount of carrying on or crying will change that.

It might be easier to understand the special character of MS if we first consider the responses we have all seen to permanent adversity. There is the 'Macho' type who grits his teeth and fights tooth and nail to overcome the problem. Grunting and snorting he says, "I can lick this thing." By definition, however, this is impossible: MS is chronic. There may be better or worse times, but it is with us for the long haul. No amount of kicking, screaming, or gnashing of teeth will eliminate its existence. This unpleasant reality is something the 'macho' type cannot accept. Instead, he is condemned to a life of perpetual frustration. He blames everyone and everything for his condition. Commonly, the medical establishment is the target of his wrath. Is it any wonder that there has been a proliferation of malpractice lawsuits?

Then, there's the person who capitulates at the first sign of adversity. The mere thought of an illness that will never get better renders this individual dumb. Whether from fear of the future or of the unknown, the result is the same, this person runs for cover at the first drop of rain. Sad to say, in so many instances this is a life needlessly wasted. A clerk at the school library where I teach took this approach. Once diagnosed with MS, she purchased a wheelchair, got in it, and spent her entire life therein. Suffice to say, I never wanted to make her acquaintance.

Between these two there is the myriad of responses that combine some of each extreme, fighting, and capitulating at different times and on different issues. Regrettably, the choice of which battles to fight is too often made neither wisely nor well. Sadly, none of these responses is entirely satisfactory to the person committed to a full life. For each lacks a guiding principle which can be applied to all situations. The macho type fails to account for the reality that MS is invariably stronger and more relentless than even the toughest and most determined individual. Like it or not, we must play by its rules. The macho type doesn't ordinarily recognize anybody's rules but his own. The pushover, for want of a better description, fails to realize that while perfect health might be out of the question, constant sickness is not the only alternative. The person who attempts to combine some of each at various times is required to decide when to be strong and when to be weak. The danger always lurks of choosing weakness when strength is appropriate, and the reverse.

My response has been to neither capitulate nor to overpower. Whether from pride or foolishness, I simply refuse to do the former, and have always been too small to entertain the idea of the latter. Fashioned by the challenge of seeing my independence slowly, relentlessly taken from me, I have learned to live independently within the confines established by MS.

Essentially, confronting MS is a psychological enterprise. I always try thinking of what I want to be, and not what I am. To be sure, I am a cripple, but that only applies to my physical being. Beyond that, I am as free as I choose to be. Being a loving husband and father, a challenging teacher, and a faithful friend are yet within my reach. Those are the things for which I want to be known. There is no reason why any of us cannot reach those levels.

Confronting MS requires staying ahead of the variety of difficulties the illness presents. Always being prepared to change the way things have always been done is crucial. As my condition is always changing, so is my response constantly changing. Teaching presents similar difficulties. My approach is almost never to lecture in class. Instead, I ask students questions about the readings assigned. Based upon their responses, I will ask a further question. This continues until, as I am wont to say, something reasonably intelligent dribbles from their lips. Knowing which question to ask next, however, requires being sufficiently astute so as to discern where the deficiencies in the student's thinking is, and which question will bring him or her closer to the correct idea. It is a constant, intellectual exercise to stay ahead of the students. Similarly, with MS, at every turn, I must be ready to adapt to the changing circumstances, for they are always changing.

There are occasions to fight and others to capitulate. The key to confronting MS is discerning properly when and how to fight, and when to concede. Even when I concede, however, I don't feel defeated. Sure, I've lost a battle, but I've not lost the war. My dignity remains unscathed because I have chosen to take a step back. The element choice is still mine.

More than ever, I depend on other people. From dressing in the morning to retiring at night, and everything in between, I require the assistance of others. Would that it were otherwise, but it isn't. No, I do not like it. Actually, I rather detest it, but I cannot avoid it. It is not something over which I have a choice. That is exactly the point. Living begins by realizing we are not completely in control any longer. Once we have accepted that sad fact, we can turn our attention towards making the most of our lives. We can concentrate our efforts on how we can make the world a better place for our having been here.

Conclusion

People ask, "How do you keep going?" They seem impressed that I am able to press on with my life. This baffles me because the alternatives are clearly worse. Would they rather that I crawled into a hole, and died? Of course not. Nevertheless, they maintain that they could never carry on in the face of adversity like mine. Nonsense! My situation is no worse than anyone else's. The only distinction is that it happens to be mine. Alexis de Tocqueville, the French aristocrat who visited America in the early 1800s, characterized my predicament beautifully. Referring to the latitude democracy enjoys, he wrote,

Providence has, in truth, drawn a predestined circle around each man beyond which he cannot pass; but within those vast limits man is strong and free…

My situation is neither better, nor worse than anyone else's. We are each born with a circle around us from our genetic makeup. MS sufferers get an additional circle. Too often, it happens to be smaller. Utilizing every square millimeter of its vast limits is my goal.

How do I keep going? The answer is simple: there is no other way. Sure, there are many alternatives, but I could not retain my self-respect if I opted for them. Is it foolish pride? Some might say so, but it is the only way I know.

Determination alone, however, is not enough. Even the most vigorous individual cannot overcome the ravages of MS. We can all cite instances of talented and athletic people who have been cut down by it. Stories of a gifted musician, a talented actress, or a prominent politician are grim reminders that all walks of life suffer. This is not to suggest that I never get angry. We are all entitled to at least that. Many people find relief in 'venting', others cry; while still others scream. Each way acts like a release valve on a pressure cooker, and we all know what happens to a pressure cooker if the steam is not released.

Arguably, the greatest challenge we face is being able to maintain our dignity despite the need for assistance. Admitting that we need help is difficult. Watching our physical abilities wither is painful and discouraging. It is something for which everyone is entitled to grieve. I've done my share. It is both logical and defensible. Pressing ahead is by no measure a joy for me, but I cannot imagine spending life indulging MS. Accommodations with the illness today are better and more extensive than they have ever been. Anything and everything necessary to make life easier should be pursued. Whether it is crutches, a cane, a catheter, a wheelchair, grab bars, a walker, or a ramp, all aids should be readily employed. There is simply no shame in needing help.

Almost unimaginable patience is required to support whatever strength I possess. Everything I do takes longer. When I want to get from here to there, I have to bide my time, plan on taking longer, and count on exerting more effort. Others get frustrated at this because they can do these things without a second thought. By contrast, I take what seems nearly forever. Thankfully, they don't get frustrated with me *per se*, but with my not being able to do what I want, when I want. I don't have the luxury of getting frustrated. If it would help to become angry, my actions would give new meaning to that word. It is not that I never get frustrated. Indeed, I dream of the day when I won't. But, frustration and anger won't change anything. Neither will they help. That realization makes being patient considerably easier. I don't delight in being patient. But, as with so many other things in my life, MS left me no choice.

Ultimately, confronting MS is a lesson in humility. Sometimes it means not being able to run with my daughters, other times it's not being able to go on the rides at the amusement park, while at others it means not walking with my wife. Accepting these limits is a constant in my life. Would that it were otherwise. Acceptance is not a single event. Rather, it is a continuing process. When first diagnosed, I vowed never to have bowel and bladder problems. The very thought of doing anything to my 'private parts' chilled my bones. Similarly, I was determined never to need a wheelchair. Today, I suffer all those problems and more. Life with MS is hardly ever stable. We must be ready to accommodate changes.

Suffering MS means being governed by a master tougher than we are. Fair enough, but who governs our master? I've never heard of MS being self-governing. Is life, then, just an accident? That seems to be the implication. No, I don't believe there are any accidents. Rather, I am convinced that there is a God who controls the universe. Why any of us gets this horrible disease is anybody's guess. Just ask a physician. They'll tell you they don't know. Nobody does. Yet there is a reason for everything. We just aren't in a position to understand it. It's as if we have a worm's eye view of the universe. We can only see our own little corner of it, but not the whole picture.

Recollections of my elders who lived through the Depression illustrate this point. They claim to understand it, but they could only see what happened to them. Their reflections are accurate, as far as they go, but they are limited to their own experience. There was considerably more to it than their view could encompass.

So, too, with MS. I can only see my case, but not the whole. Would I be a different person had I not gotten MS? No doubt, but that is irrelevant. I did get it, and my challenge is to live with it. The 'what if' question is strictly a matter of speculation. It can be asked a million times over in each of our lives. Dwelling on it is a waste of time because it changes nothing.

The illness's progress is out of our control. My challenge is to pursue a life whereby I can enrich other people's lives. Whether as a father, husband, teacher, neighbor, friend, or acquaintance, my goal is to make the world a slightly better place for my having been here. If I can make it easier for others to bear the burden of MS through this book, my life will not have been wasted.

Realizing that we cannot do everything, and reconciling ourselves to that reality is a fact of life. Sooner or later everyone is faced with this same dilemma. One of the most poignant formulations of this is by Chuck Yeager, the former WWII flying ace, test pilot, and first man to break the sound barrier. Toward the end of his autobiography, he laments that at the of age 60+, he cannot carry on as he did as a young man. No longer able to drink like a fish, party all night, or carouse like a teenager, he asks,

"How do I keep going?"

His answer:

"You back up, but you don't give up."

It is a wonderful way to approach the world.

Having MS is not an excuse for wasting one's life. Neither does it excuse self-indulgence. Granted, it has changed my life in untold ways, and many of my aspirations. No longer am I physically able to do many of the things I once could. Nevertheless, I remain the person I have always been. My goals are as dynamic as they have ever been. What defines me are the same as they have always been. Being caring and compassionate toward others is still within my grasp. So too, are they within everyone's. My deepest hope is to make life better for people with MS (and everyone around them). I want to have a favorable impact on everyone I meet, and leave a positive legacy.

0-595-25907-3